PRACTICAL ADVANCED PERIODONTAL SURGERY

PRACTICAL ADVANCED PERIODONTAL SURGERY

Serge Dibart, DMD
Professor
Clinical Director
Department of Periodontology and Oral Biology
Boston University School of Dental Medicine
Boston, MA

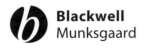

Blackwell
Munksgaard

Serge Dibart, DMD, is clinical director of the periodontal residency program at Boston University Goldman School of Graduate Dentistry.

Editorial Offices:
Blackwell Publishing Professional,
2121 State Avenue, Ames, Iowa 50014-8300, USA
  Tel: +1 515 292 0140
9600 Garsington Road, Oxford OX4 2DQ
  Tel: 01865 776868

Blackwell Publishing Asia Pty Ltd,
550 Swanston Street, Carlton South,
Victoria 3053, Australia
  Tel: +61 (0)3 9347 0300

Blackwell Wissenschafts Verlag,
Kurfürstendamm 57, 10707 Berlin, Germany
  Tel: +49 (0)30 32 79 060

Disclaimer

The contents of this work are intended to further general scientific research, understanding, and discussion only and are not intended and should not be relied upon as recommending or promoting a specific method, diagnosis, or treatment by practitioners for any particular patient. The publisher and the author make no representations or warranties with respect to the accuracy or completeness of the contents of this work and specifically disclaim all warranties, including without limitation any implied warranties of fitness for a particular purpose. In view of ongoing research, equipment modifications, changes in governmental regulations, and the constant flow of information relating to the use of medicines, equipment, and devices, the reader is urged to review and evaluate the information provided in the package insert or instructions for each medicine, equipment, or device for, among other things, any changes in the instructions or indication of usage and for added warnings and precautions. Readers should consult with a specialist where appropriate. The fact that an organization or Website is referred to in this work as a citation and/or a potential source of further information does not mean that the author or the publisher endorses the information the organization or Website may provide or recommendations it may make. Further, readers should be aware that Internet Websites listed in this work may have changed or disappeared between when this work was written and when it is read. No warranty may be created or extended by any promotional statements for this work. Neither the publisher nor the author shall be liable for any damages arising herefrom.

First published 2007 by Blackwell Munksgaard, a Blackwell Publishing Company

Library of Congress
Cataloging-in-Publication Data
  Practical advanced periodontal surgery / [edited by] Serge Dibart.
    p. ; cm.
  Includes bibliographical references and index.
  ISBN 978-0-8138-0957-1 (alk. paper)
  1. Periodontium—Surgery. I. Dibart, Serge.
[DNLM: 1. Periodontium—surgery. 2. Oral Surgical Procedures, Preprosthetic—methods. 3. Periodontics—methods. WU 240 P895 2007]

RK361.P73 2007
617.6′32—dc22
2007019841

978-0-8138-0957-1

Set by Data Management
Printed and bound by C.O.S. Printers PTE LTD

For further information on
Blackwell Publishing, visit our website:
www.blackwellpublishing.com

The last digit is the print number:
9 8 7 6 5 4 3 2

Contents

List of contributors

Serge Dibart, DMD
Professor, Department of Periodontology and Oral Biology
Director, Postgraduate Periodontal Clinic
Director, 2nd Floor Specialty Clinics
Boston University School of Dental Medicine
100 East Newton Street
Boston, MA 02118 USA
617-638-4762
sdibart@bu.edu

Nawaf J. Al-Dousari, DDS, MSD
Practice limited to prosthodontics
Armed Forces Hospital
Ministry of Defense
Kuwait Block 1 Street 16 House 2
Shamiya, Kuwait City
Kuwait
617-515-5465
nawafdds@hotmal.com

Haneen N. Bokhadoor, DDS, MSD
Practice limited to periodontics and dental implants
Bneid Al Gar Specialty Dental Center
Ministry of Health
Block 1 Street 16 House 2
Shamiya, Kuwait City
Kuwait
965-988-8028
h_bukhadhoor@hotmail.com

Jean-Pierre Dibart, MD
Rheumatology and Sport Medicine
18 Avenue de Corinthe
Marseilles, France
Dibart.jp@wanadoo.fr

Donald J. Ferguson, DMD, MSD
Professor of Orthodontics
The Anthony Gianelly Chair in Orthodontics
Department of Orthodontics and Dentofacial Orthopedics
Boston University School of Dental Medicine
100 East Newton Street
Boston, MA 02118 USA
617-414-1026
ferguson@bu.edu

Sadru Kabani, DMD, MS
Professor and Chairman
Department of Oral and Maxillofacial Pathology
Boston University School of Dental Medicine
100 East Newton Street
Boston, MA 02118 USA
617-638-5677
kabani@bu.edu

M. Gabriela Marquez, DMD, MSD
Clinical Instructor
Department of Orthodontics and Dentofacial Orthopedics
Boston University School of Dental Medicine
100 East Newton Street
Boston, MA 02118
617-792-3990
gmarquez@bu.edu

Luigi Montesani, MD, DDS
Practice limited to periodontology prosthodontics and implant dentistry
Via Lazio 6
00187 Rome
Italy
luigi@montesani.it

Steven Morgano, DMD
Professor and Director
Division of Postdoctoral Prosthodontics
Boston University School of Dental Medicine
100 East Newton Street
Boston, MA 02118 USA
617-638-5429
smorgano@bu.edu

Mani Moulazadeh, DMD
Assistant Clinical Professor and Clinical Director
Department of Endodontics
Boston University School of Dental Medicine
100 East Newton Street
Boston, MA 02118 USA
manim@bu.edu

Vikki Noonan, DMD, DMSc
Assistant Professor
Department of Oral and Maxillofacial Pathology
Boston University School of Dental Medicine
100 East Newton Street
Boston, MA 02118 USA
617-638-5677
vnoonan@bu.edu

Albert Price, DMD, MS
Associate Clinical Professor
Department of Periodontology and Oral Biology
Boston University School of Dental Medicine
100 East Newton Street
Boston, MA 02118 USA
617-638-4762
amprice@bu.edu

Ulrike Schulze-Späte, DMD, PhD
Assistant Professor
Department of Periodontology and Oral Biology
Boston University School of Dental Medicine
100 East Newton Street
Boston, MA 02118 USA
617-638-4925
uspate@bu.edu

Peyman Shahidi, DDS, MScD
Practice limited to periodontology and implant dentistry
5 Northtown Way, Suite 2101
Toronto, Ontario
M2N7A1 Canada
416-803-7626
peyshahidi@yahoo.com

Ming Fang Su, DMD, MS
Assistant Clinical Professor
Department of Periodontology and Oral Biology
Boston University School of Dental Medicine
100 East Newton Street
Boston, MA 02118 USA
617-638-4762
suming@bu.edu

M. Thomas Wilcko, DMD
Clinical Associate Professor in Periodontics
Case Western Reserve University
Private practice limited to periodontics
6074 Peach Street
Erie, PA 16509
814-868-3669
wilcko@velocity.net

William M. Wilcko, DMD, MS
Adjunct Assistant Professor of Orthodontics
Boston University
Private practice limited to orthodontics
6066 Peach Street
Erie, PA 16509
814-868-8679
fastbraces@aol.com

Thomas Van Dyke, DDS, PhD
Professor, Department of Periodontology and Oral Biology
Director, Postgraduate Periodontology
Director, Clinical Research Center
Boston University School of Dental Medicine
100 East Newton Street
Boston, MA 02118 USA
617-638-4758
tvandyke@bu.edu

Yun Po Zhang, PhD, DDS(hon)
Director
Clinical Dental Research
Colgate-Palmolive Company
909 River Road
Piscataway, NJ 08854 USA
Yun_Po_Zhang@colpal.com

Acknowledgments

I would like to thank Dean Frankl, my colleagues and students of Boston University School of Dental Medicine for their invaluable help. I would also like to thank Ms. Leila Joy Rosenthal for drawing Figures 7.32 and 7.33.

PRACTICAL ADVANCED PERIODONTAL SURGERY

Chapter 1 Introduction

Thomas Van Dyke, DDS, PhD

The specialty of periodontics has grown in the past 25 years to encompass a variety of surgical techniques that span the scope of dentistry. The advent of predictable implant placement and numerous new bone augmentation techniques has broadened the repertoire of the periodontist to a point where technical developments through research have impacted other specialties, including orthodontics, endodontics, oral and maxillofacial surgery, and prosthodontics.

In this book, *Practical Advanced Periodontal Surgery,* Dr. Serge Dibart has assembled a team of experts, mostly from the faculty of Boston University Goldman School of Dental Medicine, who have played a major role in the development of these concepts, in some cases, and their implementation, in all cases. It is arranged into 11 chapters that range from a review of the science leading up to new technologies to their implementation and the evidence backing their veracity. The contribution of periodontal concepts to orthodontics and endodontics is just an example of how modern periodontology adds to the armamentarium of all aspects of the dental profession.

The focus of this book is bone—the biology of bone and how an understanding of the basic principles of biology can be used to enhance treatment. The book begins with a review of bone biology and current understanding of wound healing. This is followed by the introduction to an exciting new area in bone biology that has been translated into effective new methods for orthodontic therapy. Dr. Donald J. Ferguson is a pioneer in this new area of accelerated osteogenic orthodontics, along with the developers of the modern concepts of the procedures, Drs. William M. Wilcko and M. Thomas Wilcko. The discovery that surgically injured bone becomes rapidly osteopenic followed by increased turnover has the potential to revolutionize a number of orthodontic procedures, which are described in this book.

The chapter on the management of periradicular periodontitis is written by a clinician-scientist, Dr. Mani Moulazadeh, who has great insight into how sound periodontal principles can have a positive impact on endodontic procedures, including apicoectomy and tooth reimplantation. Likewise, the combined impact on restoration of complex cases is addressed by a husband-and-wife team, one a periodontist (Dr. Haneen N. Bokhadoor) and one a prosthodontist (Dr. Nawaf J. Al-Dousari), and their mentor (Dr. Steven Morgano), all with particular insight into the possibilities available to practitioners in today's world. Procedures thought once to be without scientific basis and on the fringe of ethical practice have been scientifically verified, and the evidence is compelling. These

are advanced, difficult procedures, but they open up a world of possibilities for the management of difficult cases.

The final five chapters of the book are devoted to exploring the specialized needs of complex cases. The problems of inadequate vertical bone height and soft tissue defects can now be predictably addressed in most cases. In particular, the aesthetic issues of lack of papillary redevelopment between adjacent implants are addressed by established investigators in the field. Distraction osteogenesis and papilla regeneration techniques now provide a means to enhance the aesthetics of the most complicated cases.

The use of short implants in cases of minimal interarch distance or where bone augmentation is contraindicated has been controversial for some time. There have been little data available to support their use or to contraindicate their use. Investigators at Boston University School of Dental Medicine present a balanced look at the pros and cons of short implants.

Periodontal medicine has its roots in oral pathology/oral medicine. The forefathers of periodontics, physicians such as Gottlieb, Orban, and Goldman, were oral pathologists first. No book of advanced periodontal techniques would be complete without a review of the most common oral lesions that face the periodontist and their treatment, along with proper biopsy techniques. The Oral Pathology Department at Boston University School of Dental Medicine, headed by Dr. Sadru Kabani and ably supported by Dr. Vikki Noonan, is in the unique position of providing services for a large metropolitan community, Boston, and for New England. The chapter on periodontal medicine provides a state-of-the-art look at oral pathology in the periodontal practice.

Finally, we have a look to the future. Tissue-engineering techniques have been researched for a number of years, and several are ready for the clinic. Two clinician-scientists (Drs. Luigi Montesani and Ulrike Schulze-Späte) take an in-depth look at bone matrix derived from the patient's own periosteal cells that are cultivated on a polymer fleece and used for sinus floor elevation and augmentation. This is the future of periodontology; we are provided an exciting glimpse at procedures that are reality today.

Dr. Dibart is to be congratulated for bringing together the subject, the team, and the expertise to produce a most valuable compilation of advanced techniques of modern periodontics. Moreover, the content is scientific and balanced, providing a useful tool for the practitioner of advanced dentistry.

Chapter 2 Bone Physiology and Metabolism

Jean-Pierre Dibart, MD

BONE COMPOSITION

Bone consists of three types of cells and a matrix.

Cells: Osteoblasts, Osteoclasts, and Osteocytes

Osteoblasts and osteocytes (mature osteoblasts) are involved in the deposition of bone matrix. Osteoblasts are responsible for the formation of new bone; they secrete osteoid and modulate the crystallization of hydroxyapatite. Osteocytes are mature bone cells; they communicate with each other via gap junctions or canaliculi. Osteoclasts are involved in the resorption of bone tissue; they are responsible for the resorption of bone, which is necessary for its repair in case of fracture or remodeling.

Matrix: Organic and Inorganic

The organic matrix is composed of collagen fibers and a ground substance. The collagen fibers are proteins that give bone its flexibility. The ground substance is made of proteoglycans and glycosaminoglycans: keratin sulfate, chondroitin sulfate, and hyaluronic acid. These components bind cells together and are necessary for the exchange of materials.

The inorganic matrix is composed of hydroxyapatite, calcium carbonate, and calcium citrate. Hydroxyapatite gives bone its strength. Hydroxyapatite is a very hard substance; it is the main mineral component of bone and the enamel of teeth, and it contains calcium, phosphorus, oxygen, and hydrogen.

Bone is the body's major reservoir of calcium (the skeleton contains 99% of the body's calcium, as hydroxyapatite). Mature adults have about 1200 g of calcium.

BONE TYPES

There are two different types of bone:

- Cortical bone, also known as compact bone

- Trabecular bone, also known as cancellous bone

Cortical Bone

Denser and more calcified than trabecular bone, cortical bone is found in the diaphysis of long bones and in the exterior of short bones. It is also called compact bone, and it has a high resistance to bending and torsion. Osteons (Haversian system) are the predominant structures found in compact bone. Each osteon is composed of a central vascular channel, the Haversian canal, surrounded by concentric layers of matrix called lamellae. Osteocytes are found between concentric lamellae. They are connected to each other and the central canal by cytoplasmic processes through the canaliculi. Osteons are separated from each other by cement lines. The space between separate osteons is occupied by interstitial lamellae. Osteons are connected to each other and the periosteum by oblique channels called Volkmann's canals (Marieb 1998).

Trabecular Bone

Trabecular bone is more spongy than cortical bone, it has a lower calcium content and a higher turnover rate, and it is more vulnerable to bone loss. It is found at the metaphysis and diaphysis of long bones and in the interior of the short bones (spine). It is composed of bundles of short and parallel strands of bone fused together. The external layer of trabecular bone contains red bone marrow, where the production of blood cellular components takes place and where most of the arteries and veins of bone organs are located (Tortora 1989).

BONE FORMATION

Intramembranous and Endochondral Ossifications

- Intramembranous ossification: Direct replacement of connective tissue with bone (i.e., mandible and flat bones of the skull)

- Endochondral ossification: Cartilage is replaced by mineralized bone, and the bones become longer, explaining growth during childhood (i.e., femur and humerus).

Bone Remodeling

Remodeling is a sequence of activation, resorption, and formation. The bone is continuously remodeling; osteoclasts become activated and resorb the old bone, and then osteoblasts begin formation of the new bone, giving rise to the Haversian system. The mature osteoclasts resorb bone by forming a space on the matrix surface; then, the osteoids begin to mineralize, regulated by the osteoblasts.

Months later, the crystals are packed closely, and the density of the bone increases.

Remodeling is necessary to maintain bone structure after a fracture or after age-related modifications; osteoclasts resorb aging bone in order to repair damage and maintain the quality of bone and to retain calcium homeostasis.

Bone can also remodel according to stresses, such as orthodontic tooth movement, in which there is resorption on the pressure side and apposition on the traction side.

Complete rest results in accelerated bone loss, whereas weight-bearing activities are associated with bone formation. Peak bone mass is the maximum bone mass achieved by midlife. Exercise programs increase bone mass at all ages; adolescence is a particularly critical period because the velocity of bone growth doubles. When women reach menopause, bone resorption exceeds bone formation, osteoblastic activity cannot keep up with osteoclastic activity, and women begin to lose bone. This puts them at high risk for osteoporosis and fractures.

There are five stages in bone remodeling:

1. Quiescence: Resting state of the bone surface

2. Activation: Recruitment of osteoclasts to a bone surface; osteoblasts secrete collagenase

3. Resorption: Removal of bone by osteoclasts; Howship's lacunae are excavated

4. Reversal: Short phase; cement line is formed; osteoclasts stop removing bone; osteoblasts fill the defect

5. Formation: Laying down of bone; osteoblasts produce osteoid; mineralization begins; then bone is again converted to a resting surface

Bone is remodeled through the following actions:

- Osteoblasts
- Osteoclasts
- Parathyroid hormone (PTH)
- Vitamin D
- Calcitonin (CT)
- Estrogens
- Corticoids
- Growth hormone (GH)
- Thyroid hormone

Bone Remodeling and Periodontitis

After damage to the bone has occurred, the osteocytes send messages to the surface to produce preosteoblasts. They express RANK-L (receptor activator of nuclear factor [NF]-κB ligand). Preosteoclasts have receptors called RANK (receptor activator of NF-κB). RANK-ligand (RANK-L) activates these receptors, which produce mature osteoclasts. RANK, RANK-L, and osteoprotegerin (OPG) (RANK-L inhibitor) are the key factors regulating osteoclast formation in normal bone physiology. The molecular interactions of these molecules regulate osteoclast formation and bone loss in various diseases such as rheumatologic inflammatory diseases, periodontitis, or peri-implantitis (Haynes 2004). The change in the levels of these regulators plays a role in the bone loss seen in periodontitis. Significantly higher levels of RANK-L protein were found to be expressed in the periodontally affected tissues, whereas OPG protein levels are lower. RANK-L protein is associated with lymphocytes and macrophages; many leukocytes expressing messenger RNA (mRNA) are observed in periodontitis tissues (Crotti et al. 2003). RANK-L is a TNF (tumor necrosis factor) receptor–related protein and a major factor for osteoclast differentiation and activation. The levels of RANK-L mRNA are higher in advanced periodontitis; although the levels of OPG mRNA are lower in advanced and moderate periodontitis, the ratio of RANK-L to OPG mRNA is increased in periodontitis. RANK-L mRNA is expressed in proliferating epithelium and in inflammatory cells, mainly lymphocytes and macrophages. Upregulation of RANK-L mRNA is associated with the activation of osteoclastic bone destruction in periodontitis (Liu et al. 2003).

Markers of Bone Formation

Markers of bone formation measure osteoblastic activity: osteocalcin, P1NP (N-terminal propeptide of type 1 procollagen), and bone-specific alkaline phosphatase (BALP).

Markers of Bone Resorption

These markers measure osteoclastic activity: deoxypyridinoline (DPD), pyridinoline and associated peptides, NTX (cross-linked N-terminal telopeptide of type I collagen), and CTX I (cross-linked C-terminal telopeptide of type I collagen) generated from bone by osteoclasts as a degradation product of type I collagen and released into circulation.

Vitamin C

This vitamin is necessary for the osteocytes to form collagen; in the case of vitamin C deficiency, collagen formation is decreased, and so is the thickness of the bone cortex.

Vitamin D

It has an important role in calcium absorption. The two major forms involved in humans are vitamin D_2 (ergocalciferol) and vitamin D_3 (cholecalciferol). 1,25-Dihydroxy-vitamin D_3 [1,25-(OH)2 vitamin D_3] is produced by metabolism in the liver and the kidneys. It is the most active form of vitamin D, and it increases calcium absorption from the intestines. Conversion into the active metabolite 1,25-(OH)2 vitamin D_3 from its precursor is affected by cytochrome P450 enzymes in the liver and the kidneys. This is tightly regulated by the plasma levels of calcium, phosphate, PTH, and 1,25-(OH)2 vitamin D_3 itself (Tissandie et al. 2006). It affects the kidneys and the intestines and stimulates the mineralization of bone. Ultraviolet irradiation from the sunlight to the skin will also affect the production of vitamins D_2 and D_3.

Genetic polymorphisms in the vitamin D receptor (*VDR*) gene are associated with parameters of bone homeostasis and with osteoporosis and rapid bone resorption. Interestingly, some authors have found *VDR* polymorphism to be associated with localized aggressive periodontal disease (Hennig et al. 1999)

Childhood vitamin D deficiency syndrome is called rickets: unmineralized osteoid accumulates, and the bone formed is weak and can lead to permanent deformities of the skeleton. In adulthood, the absence of adequate amounts of vitamin D leads to osteomalacia: decalcification of bone occurs by defective mineralization of newly formed bone matrix.

What are the sources of vitamin D? Only a few foods contain appreciable amounts of vitamin D—fish liver, fish (i.e., salmon, mackerel, tuna, sardines), eggs, liver, butter, and Shiitake mushrooms.

Vitamin K

This vitamin is required for the production of osteocalcin (a protein produced by the osteoblasts); a good vitamin K status is necessary to prevent osteoporosis. Vitamin K is found in green leafy vegetables.

Calcitonin

This is a hormone secreted by the thyroid gland. Its effects are opposite those of the PTH (lowering of blood calcium). Calcitonin inhibits matrix resorption by inhibiting osteoclast activity; it reverses hypercalcemia.

Parathyroid Hormone

PTH is a hormone produced by the parathyroid glands. It increases ionized blood calcium levels. The fall in ionized blood calcium causes the release of PTH and vitamin D. PTH stimulates osteoclast activity, and calcium is released from the bone. PTH causes resorption of bone, calcium absorption from the kidneys, and synthesis of active vitamin D. Bone calcium mobilization is due to the transfer of calcium ions from hydroxyapatite to blood, to ensure calcium homeostasis.

PTH activates and increases the number of osteoclasts, causing resorption of the bone matrix. PTH also acts on the kidneys to decrease urinary calcium.

Hyperparathyroidism causes increased bone resorption.

Osteoprotegerin

OPG is an inhibitor of bone resorption and is involved in bone density regulation. High levels cause the development of dense bone. OPG blocks the differentiation of osteoclasts and impairs bone resorption.

Low-Density Lipoprotein Receptor–Related Proteins

Recent analyses revealed a new signaling pathway involved in the regulation of osteoblastic cells and the acquisition of peak bone mass. Wnts are soluble glycoproteins that engage receptor complexes composed of low-density lipoprotein receptor–related proteins Lrp 5 and 6 and Frizzled proteins. The loss of function of Lrp 5 causes a decrease in bone formation, and Lrp 5 mutations are associated with high bone mass diseases. These mutations influence the Wnt-beta-catenin canonical pathway that increases bone mass through a large number of mechanisms.

Osteoporosis

Osteoporosis means "porous bone." Calcium deficiency leads to decalcification of bones and aggravated fracture risks (especially vertebrae, hip, and forearm). Hyperparathyroidism can also cause decalcification. Androgens and estrogens (especially before menopause), on the other hand, stimulate bone formation.

Osteoporosis is characterized by low bone mass and microarchitectural deterioration due to decreased bone formation and increased bone resorption; this phenomenon leads to increased bone fragility and fracture. As we age, bone resorption exceeds bone formation and the severe loss of bone mass results in gaps in the bone structure, leading to fractures (hip, spine, and wrist being the most common).

Bone strength is also determined by another important element, which is the trabecular microstructure. In estrogen deficiency, resorption cavities are too deep and the trabeculae are not well connected, resulting in increased bone fragility.

In women after age 30, bone resorption exceeds bone formation and bone mass decreases slowly. After menopause, because of a decrease in estrogen levels, bone loss is accelerated. Peak bone density is lower in females than in males, and bone mineral status depends on peak bone mass achieved before the age of 30. Optimizing peak bone mass, especially in children and adolescents, between the ages of 10 to 18, is important in reducing the future risk of osteoporosis.

Although most of the variance in peak bone mass is considered to be genetic, bone mineral density is higher with sufficient consumption of calcium, fruits, and vegetables. Calcium-rich foods include dairy products, cereals, nuts, seeds, dried fruits, mineral water, and green-leafed vegetables.

Risk factors include the following:

- Female patients after menopause or age over 60
- First-degree female relative with osteoporosis or fracture
- Personal history of nontraumatic fracture
- Low body mass index (BMI) (<19 kg/m^2)
- Anorexia-amenorrhea episodes
- Excessive sports participation
- Prolonged use of cortisone
- Early menopause before age 40, natural or surgically induced
- Smoking
- Excessive alcohol intake
- Sedentary lifestyle
- Excessive caffeine or salt intake
- Low calcium intake
- Thyroid hormone or PTH abnormalities
- Hypercortisolism
- Prevalent radiographic vertebral fracture

BONE DENSITY MEASURING TECHNIQUES

DEXA: Dual Energy X-ray Absorptiometry (Bone Densitometry)

In DEXA, an x-ray with two energy peaks is sent through the bones. One is absorbed by the soft tissues, and the other is absorbed by the bones; through subtraction, bone mineral density (BMD) is measured. This is the most widely used method to measure bone density and provides whole-body scans and detailed measurements of the spine (lumbar spine), the hip (femoral neck), and the forearm (wrist).

The World Health Organization definition of *osteoporosis* is based on BMD expressed as T scores and Z scores:

- T score is the comparison with the bone density of young people.
- Z score is the comparison with the bone density of age peers.
- A T score superior to –2.5 standard deviation is the definition of *osteoporosis*. The WHO based the diagnosis of postmenopausal osteoporosis on the presence of a BMD T-score that is 2.5 standard deviations or more below the mean for young women.
- A T score between –1 and –2.5 standard deviations is the definition of *osteopenia*.

Quantitative Ultrasound

Quantitative ultrasound (QUS) is a radiation-free reliable technique to evaluate skeletal status. Three parameters are measured: broadband ultrasound attenuation (BUA), speed of sound (SOS), and stiffness index (SI).

This is a technique performed with use of the calcaneous or radial bone; it measures the bone mass on the basis of the bone SOS.

Quantitative Computed Tomography

Quantitative computed tomography (QCT) provides three-dimensional BMD of trabecular and cortical components. It is also used to analyze trabecular microstructure.

This technique measures an imaged slice of the forearm or the leg; it can be used to measure bone size and the width of cortical and trabecular bone. It provides a volumetric density of bone. It can also measure the volume and content of calcium hydroxyapatite.

Cone Beam Computed Tomography

This technique offers a significant advantage because of its three-dimensional capability for osseous defects detection (Misch et al. 2006).

Fractal Analysis of Bone Texture

The analysis of bone texture based on fractal mathematics when applied to bone images on plain radiographs can be considered as a reflection of trabecular bone microarchitecture.

IMPLICATIONS FOR DENTAL TREATMENTS

Osteonecrosis of the Jaws

Bisphosphonates are used in treatment of cancers and osteoporosis; as a side effect, they may cause jaw necrosis. These necroses mostly appear after administration of amino-bisphosphonates. They are treated by resection of necrotic bone, and repeated surgical interventions are required. The management is difficult and includes surgical procedures and antibiotic therapy (Eckert et al. 2007).

Bisphosphonates somehow cause cell death in the jawbone, which makes it prone to chronic infection; the reduced resorptive ability of bone due to bisphosphonates hinders the formation of a fresh bone surface for reestablishment of bone cell coverage (Aspenberg 2006).

The clinical symptoms of jaw necrosis are swelling, exudation, loosening of teeth, and pain. The radiographs show persisting tooth sockets after extractions and radiolucency, sequestra, or fracture. Risk factors are as follows:

- Intravenous or long-term bisphosphonate therapy (over 3 years of oral use, over 1 year of intravenous use)
- Chemotherapy
- Radiation
- Corticoids
- Age
- Underlying malignant disease
- Oral infection

Bisphosphonate-associated osteonecrosis is characterized by the unexpected appearance of necrotic bone. Osteonecrosis can develop spontaneously or after an invasive surgical procedure such as dental extraction. Symptoms can mimic routine dental problems such as decay or periodontal disease. Risk factors are intravenous bisphosphonate therapy, duration of treatment, age greater than 60 years, myeloma, and history of recent dental extraction (Migliorati et al. 2006).

Before bisphosphonate therapy is started, infections should be treated and risk of injuries to the mucosa should be reduced. Regular dental recall is recommended, for the prevention of infection combined with a follow-up of removable denture for possible ulcerations. Conservative treatment measures are preferred; surgery is carried out nontraumatically using sterile techniques, appropriate oral disinfectant, and antibiotic prophylaxis until the day of suture removal. For patients following bisphosphonate therapy, the indications for dental implants should be very strict; in case of the osteonecrosis, dental implants are contraindicated (Piesold et al. 2006).

Early diagnosis is important; it can make a difference in the outcome of the disease. Technetium 99m-methylene diphosphonate (MDP) three-phase bone scan can be used as a screening test to detect subclinical osteonecrosis. Computed tomography (CT) and magnetic resonance imaging (MRI) are useful in defining the features and extent of lesions. Radiography and CT display osteolytic lesions with the involvement of cortical bone, and MRI shows the edema of soft tissue. ^{99m}Tc-MDP three-phase bone scan is the most sensitive tool to detect necrosis at an early stage (Chiandusi et al. 2006).

The mandible is more commonly affected than the maxilla and 60% of cases are preceded by a dental surgical procedure. Oversuppression of bone turnover is the primary mechanism of necrosis, and there may be comorbid factors. All sites of jaw infection should be eliminated before bisphosphonate therapy in at-risk patients. Conservative debridement, pain control, infection management, use of antimicrobial rinses, and withdrawal of bisphosphonate are preferable to aggressive surgical measures (Woo et al. 2006).

Dental Implants

Bone quality and its presurgical assessment are important for long-term implant prognosis; the implant length and type can also influence bone strain, especially in low-density bone (Tada et al. 2003).

The Process of Osseointegration

In the early bone response to the implant, the first tissue that comes in contact with the implant is the blood clot with platelets and fibrin. During the first days, preosteoblasts and osteoblasts adhere to the implant surface covered by an afibrillar calcified layer to produce osteoid tissue; within a few days, a woven bone and then a reparative trabecular bone are present at the junction between the implant and the bone. Trabecular bone is gradually substituted by a mature lamellar bone, which characterizes osseointegration (Marco et al. 2005).

Osseointegration is a dynamic process: in the establishment phase, there is an interplay between bone resorption in contact regions and bone formation in contact-free areas. During the maintenance phase, osseointegration is secured through continuous remodeling and adaptation to function (Berglundh et al. 2003).

The process of osseointegration is a reliable type of cement-free anchorage for prosthetic tissue substitutes and bone, with a direct contact between living bone and implant (Albrektsson et al. 1981).

It is important to note that senile and postmenopausal osteoporosis have important consequences for the success of endosseous dental implants, for primary stability, biological fixation, and final osseointegration.

Smokers are also at risk. Bone resorption is altered in smokers; there are differences between the amounts of pyridinoline around the teeth of nonsmokers and smokers. Smokers have a higher level of pyridinoline than do nonsmokers in the gingival crevicular fluid of implants, suggesting that smoking may affect implant success (Oates et al. 2004).

Bone-Stimulating Factors

A bone differentiation factor can stimulate bone formation in peri-implant bone defects. Bone morphogenetic proteins (recombinant human bone morphogenetic protein-2 [rhBMP-2]) can be used to stimulate bone growth around and onto the surface of endosseous dental implants, placed in sites with extended osseous defects (Cochran et al. 1999). Recombinant human osteogenic protein-1 (rhOP-1) accelerates the healing of extraction defects and the osseointegration of implants. New bone formation can be induced around and adjacent to a dental implant with a recombinantly produced bone inductive protein (Cook et al. 1995).

Enamel matrix derivative (EMD) may contribute to inducing osteoblast growth and differentiation by helping create a favorable osteogenic microenvironment (reducing RANK-L release and enhancing osteoprotegerin production) (Galli et al. 2006). Amelogenins, EMDs, have a stimulatory effect on mesenchymal cells and tissues and on the regeneration of alveolar bone. They cause an increase in alkaline phosphatase activity and an increased expression of osteocalcin and type I collagen. Researchers found similarities between EMDs and PTH on human osteoblasts (Reseland et al. 2006).

Periodontitis

Patients with aggressive periodontitis share periodontal and hematological characteristics with patients with rheumatoid arthritis or juvenile idiopathic arthritis. Patients with rheumatoid arthritis have a higher percentage of sites with probing depth greater than 4 mm, clinical attachment loss greater than 2 mm, and alveolar bone loss greater than 2 mm. The percentage of sites with clinical attachment loss is correlated with the levels of serum rheumatoid factor (Havemose-Poulsen et al. 2006).

For patients with primary Sjögren syndrome, complications of periodontitis such as bleeding, gingival hypertrophy, and pockets are not improved with better oral hygiene. This phenomenon is associated with high levels of B-cell activating factor (BAFF) in the saliva; the levels of BAFF correlate with the periodontal pocket depth. The known effect of B cells in periodontitis is partly mediated by salivary BAFF in patients with primary Sjögren syndrome (Pers et al. 2005).

Mandibular Osteoporosis

There are relationships between oral bone loss and osteoporosis. There is a positive correlation between systemic bone mass and oral bone mass (Jeffcoat 2005).

Osteoporosis is a systemic disease in which the skeletal condition is characterized by a decreased mass of normally mineralized bone. Alveolar processes provide the bony framework for tooth support; the decline of skeletal mass is correlated with an increased risk of oral bone loss and has a negative effect on tooth stability. Aging and estrogen depletion have a negative influence on tooth retention and residual alveolar crest preservation (Sanfilippo & Bianchi 2003).

Pixel intensity values and fractal dimensions on radiographic panoramic images are useful in detecting changes in the osteoporotic mandibular cancellous bone (Tosoni et al. 2006). The measurement of mandibular alveolar bone mineral density, in postmenopausal women with periodontal disease, shows age-related decrease of alveolar BMD, calcaneus SOS, and vertebral BMD. There are significant correlations between alveolar BMD, calcaneus SOS, and vertebral BMD (Takaishi et al. 2005).

REFERENCES

Albrektsson, T., P.I. Branemark, H.A. Hansson, and J. Lindstrom. 1981. Osseointegrated titanium implants. Requirements for ensuring a long-lasting, direct bone-to-implant anchorage in man. Acta Orthop. Scand. 52(2):155–170.

Aspenberg, P. 2006. Osteonecrosis: what does it mean? One condition partly caused by bisphosphonates—or another one, preferably treated with them? Acta Orthop. 77(5):693–694.

Berglundh, T., I. Abrahamsson, N.P. Lang, and J. Lindhe. 2003. De novo alveolar bone formation adjacent to endosseous implants. Clin. Oral Implants Res. 14(3):251–262.

Chiandusi, S., M. Biasotto, F. Dore, F. Cavalli, M.A. Cova, and R. Di Lenarda. 2006. Clinical and diagnostic imaging of bisphosphonate-associated osteonecrosis of the jaws. Dentomaxillofac. Radiol. 35(4):236–243.

Cochran, D., R. Schenk, D. Buser, J.M. Wozney, and A.A. Jones. 1999. Recombinant human bone morphogenetic protein-2 stimulation of bone formation around endosseous dental implants. J. Periodontol. 70(2):139–150.

Cook, S.D., S.L. Salkeld, and D.C. Rueger. 1995. Evaluation of recombinant human osteogenic protein-1 (rhOP-1) placed with dental implants in fresh extraction sites. J. Oral Implantol. 21(4):281–289.

Crotti, T., M.D. Smith, R. Hirsch, S. Soukoulis, H. Weedon, M. Capone, M.J. Ahern, and D. Haynes. 2003. Receptor activator NF kappaB ligand (RANKL) and osteoprotegerin (OPG) protein expression in periodontitis. J. Periodont. Res. 38(4):380–387.

Eckert, A.W., P. Maurer, L. Meyer, M.S. Kriwalsky, R. Rohrberg, D. Schneider, U. Bilkenroth, and J. Schubert. 2007. Bisphosphonate-related jaw necrosis—severe complication in maxillofacial surgery. Cancer Treat. Rev. In press.

Galli, C., G.M. Macaluso, S. Guizzardi, R. Vescovini, M. Passeri, and G. Passeri. 2006. Osteoprotegerin and receptor activator of nuclear factor-kappa B ligand modulation by enamel matrix derivative in human alveolar osteoblasts. J. Periodontol. 77(7):1223–1228.

Havemose-Poulsen, A., J. Westergaard, K. Stoltze, H. Skjodt, B. Danneskiold-Samsoe, H. Locht, K. Bendtzen, and P. Holmstrup. 2006. Periodontal and hematological characteristics associated with aggressive periodontitis, juvenile idiopathic arthritis, and rheumatoid arthritis. J. Periodontol. 77(2):280–288.

Haynes, D.R. 2004. Bone lysis and inflammation. Inflamm. Res. 53(11): 596–600.

Hennig, B.J., J.M. Parkhill, I.L. Chapple, P.A. Heasman, and J.J. Taylor. 1999. Association of a vitamin D receptor gene polymorphism with localized early-onset periodontal diseases. J. Periodontol. 70(9):1032–1038.

Jeffcoat, M. 2005. The association between osteoporosis and oral bone loss. J. Periodontol. 76(11 Suppl):2125–2132.

Liu, D., J.K. Xu, L. Figliomeni, L. Huang, N.J. Pavlos, M. Rogers, A. Tan, P. Price, and M.H. Zheng. 2003. Expression of RANKL and OPG mRNA in periodontal disease: possible involvement in bone destruction. Int. J. Mol. Med. 11(1):17–21.

Marco, F., F. Milena, G. Gianluca, and O. Vittoria. 2005. Peri-implant osteogenesis in health and osteoporosis. Micron 36(7–8):630–644.

Marieb, E.N. (1998). *Human Anatomy & Physiology*, 4th ed. Benjamin/ Cummings Science Publishing, Menlo Park, Calif.

Migliorati, C.A., M.A. Siegel, and L.S. Elting. 2006. Bisphosphonate-associated osteonecrosis: a long-term complication of bisphosphonate treatment. *Lancet Oncol.* 7(6):508–514.

Misch, K.A., E.S. Yi, and D.P. Sarment. 2006. Accuracy of cone beam computed tomography for periodontal defect measurements. *J. Periodontol.* 77(7):1261–1266.

Oates, T.W., D. Caraway, and J. Jones. 2004. Relation between smoking and biomarkers of bone resorption associated with dental endosseous implants. *Implant Dent.* 13(4):352–357.

Pers, J.O., F. d'Arbonneau, V. Devauchelle-Pensec, A. Saraux, Y.L. Pennec, and P. Youinou. 2005. Is periodontal disease mediated by salivary BAFF in Sjogren's syndrome? *Arthrit. Rheum.* 52(8): 2411–2414.

Piesold, J.U., B. Al Nawas, and K.A. Grotz. 2006. Osteonecrosis of the jaws by long term therapy with bisphosphonates. *Mund Kiefer Gesichtschir.* 10(5):287–300.

Reseland, J.E., S. Reppe, A.M. Larsen, H.S. Berner, F.P. Reinholt, K.M. Gautvik, I. Slaby, and S.P. Lyngstadaas. 2006. The effect of enamel matrix derivative on gene expression in osteoblasts. *Eur. J. Oral Sci.* 114(Suppl 1):205–211.

Sanfilippo, F., and A.E. Bianchi. 2003. Osteoporosis: the effect on maxillary bone resorption and therapeutic possibilities by means of implant prostheses—a literature review and clinical considerations. *Int. J. Periodont. Restor. Dent.* 23(5):447–457.

Tada, S., R. Stegaroiu, E. Kitamura, O. Miyakawa, and H. Kusakari. 2003. Influence of implant design and bone quality on stress/strain distribution in bone around implants: a 3-dimensional finite element analysis. *Int. J. Oral Maxillofac. Implants* 18(3):357–368.

Takaishi, Y., Y. Okamoto, T. Ikeo, H. Morii, M. Takeda, K. Hide, T. Arai, and K. Nonaka. 2005. Correlations between periodontitis and loss of mandibular bone in relation to systemic bone changes in postmenopausal Japanese women. *Osteoporosis Int.* 16(12): 1875–1882.

Tissandie, E., Y. Gueguen, J.M. Lobaccaro, F. Paquet, J. Aigueperse, and M. Souidi. 2006. Effects of depleted uranium after short-term exposure on vitamin D metabolism in rat. *Arch. Toxicol.* 80(8): 473–480.

Tortora, G.J. (1989). *Principles of Human Anatomy*, 5th ed. Harper & Row, New York.

Tosoni, G.M., A.G. Lurie, A.E. Cowan, and J.A. Burleson. 2006. Pixel intensity and fractal analyses: detecting osteoporosis in perimenopausal and postmenopausal women by using digital panoramic images. *Oral Surg. Oral Med. Oral Pathol. Oral Radiol. Endod.* 102(2):235–241.

Woo, S.B., J.W. Hellstein, and J.R. Kalmar. 2006. Narrative [corrected] review: bisphosphonates and osteonecrosis of the jaws. *Ann. Intern. Med.* 144(10):753–761.

Chapter 3 The Wound-Healing Process

Albert Price, DMD, MS

ANATOMIC REVIEW (EMPHASIS ON VASCULAR SUPPLY)

Knowledge of local anatomy and the physiology of healing tissues is the *sine qua non* of the surgeon's ability to achieve stable results. A practical review of regional and periodontal anatomy needs to consider both the macro and micro levels that have a direct effect on surgical care. The basic process and current knowledge of wound healing are reviewed. The general principles involved are then applied to periodontal surgery procedures and utilization of dental implants. Throughout this exploration, several themes are reinforced:

1. For parts to heal, they must be *stabilized* relative to each other. Lack of mobility allows reconnection of extracellular matrix and vascular supply between the wound interfaces and eventually leads to an ordered stable repair or regeneration.

2. Understanding *microvascular patterns* and *local preservation* is the key to minimal morbidity. Poorly designed flaps can lead to soft tissue necrosis and subsequent bone loss or sequestration if the bone component is dependent on the soft tissue supply.

3. *Hard* and *soft tissue architecture* influences *microvascular architecture.* The relative physical dimensions and quality of tissue content determine blood vessel location and volume. The latter is a paraphrase of the term *biotype.* Recognition of biotype is part of treatment planning.

Constant reflection on these three themes will maximize the application to everyday surgical problems.

THE TISSUES AND THEIR VASCULAR SUPPLY

While the facial artery has some supplementary supply to the lips and nose and a submental branch supplies the sublingual gland, the major blood supply to the oral structures is through the tributaries of the maxillary artery and its regional divisions: the mandibular, the pterygoid (in the infratemporal fossa), and the pterygopalatine (in the sphenopalatine fossa) (Woodburne 1965) (Fig. 3.1).

The mandibular branches of the maxillary artery are the lingual, mylohyoid, and inferior alveolar, which enters the mandibular foramen and distributes to bone, teeth, and periodontal ligament and, before spreading out to supply the anterior teeth, emerges in a reverse curl through the mental foramen.

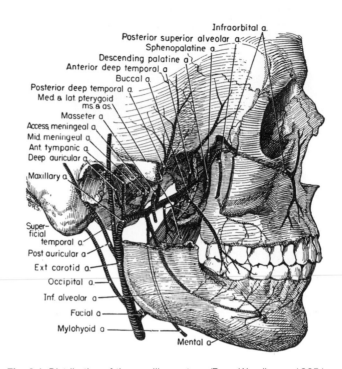

Fig. 3.1 Distribution of the maxillary artery. (From Woodburne 1965.)

The pterygoid division supplies muscles with the buccinator branch, also supplying the cheek mucosa.

The pterygopalatine division courses through the pterygopalatine fossa and sends four major branches to the posterior superior alveolar, descending palatine, infraorbital, and sphenopalatine. The posterior superior alveolar enters the distal of the maxillary tuberosity and supplies the teeth, gingiva, and maxillary sinus. The descending palatine exits through the greater palatine foramen apical to the molars and courses forward along the palatal vault (Fig. 3.2), supplying glands and mucosa until it reaches the incisive canal, where it anastomoses with the incisive branch of the sphenopalatine artery. The infraorbital passes medial through the floor of the orbit with branches to the mid and anterior incisive areas, the maxillary sinus, and the lacrimal duct and then exits through the infraorbital notch to the face. The sphenopalatine rises to the roof of the nose and then distributes forward and down to the lateral nasal wall (common with the medial wall of maxillary sinus) and medially along the vomer groove to the incisive canal, where it de-

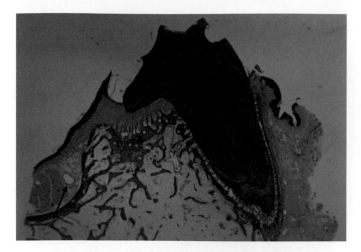

Fig. 3.2 Palatal artery–greater palatine artery (*arrow*).

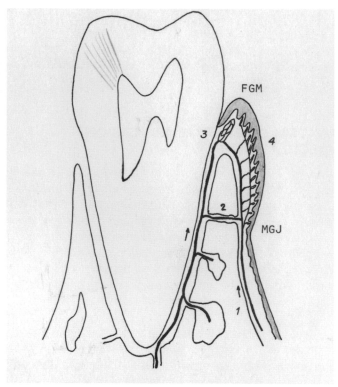

Fig. 3.3 Normal vascular supply. 1, Periosteal supply; 2, vessels from bone; 3, periodontal ligament supply to crest; 4, papillary loops.

scends to merge with the incisive branch of the greater palatine (Woodburne 1965) (see Fig. 3.1).

ALVEOLAR AND BASAL BONE

The general pattern of flow is from distal to mesial with respect to the alveolar structures. The bone compartment of the basal and alveolar bone is supplied from within their defining cortical plates (i.e., from inside-out). If teeth are present, they are surrounded by a cortical socket of woven bone that has numerous perforations connecting the marrow with the periodontal ligament (PDL) net. This PDL net is also supplied from the apical where vessels enter the tooth pulp canal. The flow of the PDL net is outward to the attached gingiva (Folke 1965, Folkman and Klagsbrun 1987) (Fig. 3.3).

Terminology

Clarification of bone terminology is necessary to discuss terms that are useful clinically. Bone has two compartments: a hard mineralized component and a soft inner marrow space. Throughout the body, these two components are arranged in various ways and proportions—the *local bony architecture*. The interface between the internal soft tissue *(marrow)* and the external investing soft tissues is occupied by a quiescent lining layer—the *endosteum* and *periosteum,* respectively. Structurally, the thick mineralized layers that define the bone's shape or line the major inclusions (major vessel channels and tooth sockets; Figs. 3.4 and 3.5) are referred to as *compact* or *cortical bone.* The inner compartment or marrow space is cross-braced by mineralized struts of various thicknesses, the *trabeculae.* These trabeculae divide the space into cells of various sizes and are termed *cancellous bone* (Figs. 3.4 and 3.5).

In clinical discourse, the word *density* is often misapplied in describing bone structure. Both cortical layers and trabeculae have a fairly uniform mineral density. What is more relevant to

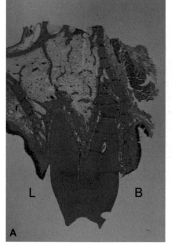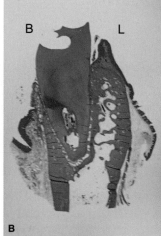

Fig. 3.4 Internal architecture. **A,** Maxillary bicuspid. **B,** Mandibular first bicuspid. Note different cortex and trabecular thicknesses. B, buccal area; L, lingual area.

surgery is the internal and external microarchitecture—the three-dimensional size and arrangement of these compact and cancellous layers. As can be seen in the representative pictures, the size and distribution of trabeculae and cortical layers vary considerably from one location to another (see

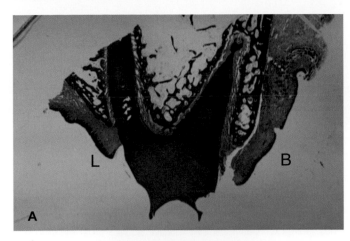

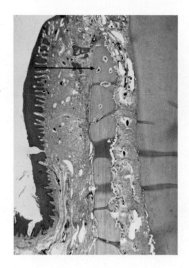

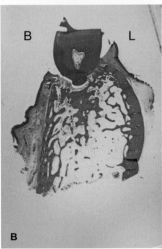

Fig. 3.5 Internal architecture of furcation area of first molars. **A,** Maxillary first molar. **B,** Mandibular first molar. Note differences in cortex and trabecular dimensions at maxillary versus mandibular sites. B, buccal area; L, lingual area.

Fig. 3.6 Small perfused vessels in very thin buccal plate (*arrow*). Note: Bone cells cannot live more than 0.1 to 0.2 mm from the blood supply.

Figs. 3.4 and 3.5). Cortical layers form the outer borders of the facial and lingual (palatal) plates of the alveolar and basal bone and the lining of the tooth sockets. Cortex is also present at the borders of the sinus, nose, and vascular channels—the *inferior alveolar canal, mental foramen,* and *incisal canal.*

Cortical by definition is "without marrow" but "not without a vasculature." These cortical parts of bone are densely calcified collagen layers with self-entrapped osteoblasts *(osteocytes).* These enclosed cells maintain contact with each other and outside nutritional sources through tiny cytoplasmic extensions within channels called *canaliculi.* There is a critical distance from the vasculature to these canals beyond which these cells cannot survive (0.1 to 0.2 mm) (Ham 1965). Even in the cortical bone, small vascular channels perfuse the structure (Fig. 3.6). Marrow of cancellous bone can be fibrous or fatty, or a combination, and it has more varied vascular supply as well as cells with regenerative potential.

The spatial position of teeth in the alveolar housing requires consideration because it influences the vascular distribution in the adjacent bone mass. In most cases, the teeth are set toward the buccal limits of their confining bone "house," commonly called the *alveolar bone.* This results in a very thin, entirely cortical bone plate on the buccal (Fig. 3.6), while the lingual limits can have a thicker compact surface with marrow between it and the alveolus as the structure extends apically. The vascular supply to these thin buccal plates, because there is no marrow supply, is limited to diffusion from the buccal through the investing mucosal tissues and internally from the PDL. (Note in Fig. 3.6 that resorption is proceeding on the PDL side of the thin buccal plate, which has had a full-thickness flap reflected.) In interproximal, lingual, and furcal areas, the internal marrow supply supplements the PDL.

The Maxilla and Mandible

The maxilla and mandible have major differences in their bony architecture, and this is reflected in the pattern of their vascular supply. The maxilla is of lighter construction and interfaces with other cranial structures of intramembranous origin. The mandible is heavy, more self-contained, and closer to the endochondral embryology of the other long bones.

In the maxilla, as noted, the major supply of blood comes from the pterygopalatine division of the maxillary artery. In the case of the maxillary sinus, the blood flow is from the superior alveolar, infraorbital, and sphenopalatine arteries. A major arterial branch is occasionally found running anterior to posterior along the lateral wall of the sinus. This artery may fall within the marrow of the antral wall if the wall is thick enough,

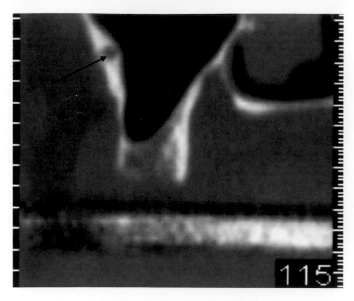

Fig. 3.7 CT scan showing artery in buccal wall of sinus (*arrow*).

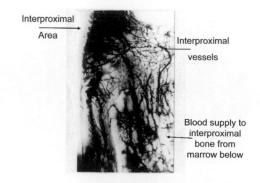

Fig. 3.8 Partial-thickness flap at 14 days showing extensive arborization and density of vessels in interproximal papilla supplied by interdental arteries. Interproximal area: papillary vascular supply is from interproximal area.

or sometimes within the periosteal layer of the sinus lining immediately inside (Fig. 3.7).

The mandibular supply is less diffuse than the maxillary, with major vessels entering through the mandibular foramen as the inferior alveolar and then spreading out confined within the core of the mandible. The flow is from the distal through the marrow and outward through the PDL. Added supplies nourish the external surfaces of the mandible, but there are few interconnections from outside with inward vessel distribution, and there are few Volkman-type vessels running from inside out through the cortex. The mandibular lingual surface has the thinnest mucosa and heaviest bone with minimal interconnection between marrow and investing soft tissue (see Fig. 3.4). Interdental and furcal subdivisions of the alveolar bone have marrow supply (Fig. 3.8).

In macroview, the external surface of the alveolar bone is sculpted with a variety of eminences and depressions, some of which shelter vital glands. Of particular importance in the maxillary arch are the central incisal and cuspid eminence and the adjacent incisal fossa (above the lateral) and cuspid fossa (over the first bicuspid). In the lower arch, there are lingual concavities beneath the lower cuspid (sublingual gland) and below the lower molars, where the mylohyoid muscle inserts (the submandibular gland is apical to this).

The alveolar bone (tooth socket) is nourished by multiple perforations of vessels from the marrow through the cortical plates and from the PDL, which has some interconnection at the crest with the gingival supply. Flow is from apical and adjacent bone marrow into the PDL and then coronally toward the alveolar socket crest, where it interconnects with the mucosal supply.

NORMAL SOFT CONNECTIVE TISSUES

The soft connective tissues of the mucosa and gingiva have structural variation, which influences vascular supply. There are three patterns to consider: the palatal, the lingual of the mandibular teeth, and the buccal of both arches.

In the palate, the thick, dense collagenous lamina propria of the anterior and bicuspid areas continues into the periosteum with some fat content, while in the molar region, a submucosa of fat and glandular tissue is present. The main vascular supply is from the greater palatine artery, which emanates from the posterior palatine canal and spreads forward, distributing supply to the palatal mucosa and ending with connection to the incisal canal branch of the sphenopalatine artery.

On the lingual of the mandibular teeth, the thin mucosal connective tissues reflect into a vestibule with loose attachment to underlying muscle. The lingual artery distributes upward to the muscles, lingual mucosa of the floor, and sublingual and submandibular glands. It should be noted that the lingual and mylohyoid nerves distribute along the inferior surface of the mylohyoid, having separated from the inferior alveolar before it enters the mandibular foramen.

The buccal connective tissue of both arches is of greater interest from a number of surgical perspectives. The buccal is juxtaposed to very thin cortical plates over the teeth, and the influence of biotype is more relevant to surgical disruption of its vascular supply.

In the marginal attached gingiva, the lamina propria has a fiber content of thick heavy collagen. (There is no lamina propria.) These densely woven bundles are physically attached to the cementum (supracrestal) between teeth (interdental) and around teeth (circumferential) and to the underlying bone (Sharpey's fibers).

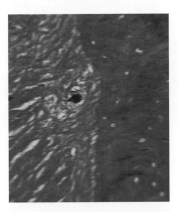

Fig. 3.9 Periosteum in attached gingival zone: dense Sharpey's fiber insertion.

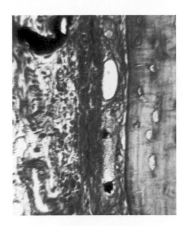

Fig. 3.11 Periosteum in mucosal zone: fibers run parallel to surface.

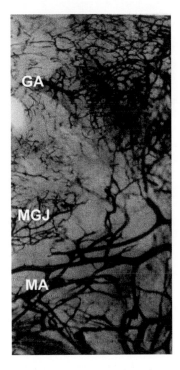

Fig. 3.10 Full-thickness flap at 7 days. Periosteal zone of connective tissue was stripped from inner surface of flap. Note the differences in vessel size and complexity of mucosa versus gingival (view from buccal). GA, gingival area; MGJ, mucogingival junction; MA, mucosal area. The larger vessels are visible.

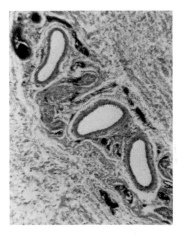

Fig. 3.12 Large arteries and veins in mucosal area.

This heavy fiber connection continues to the mucogingival junction and is the "attachment" of the attached gingiva (Fig. 3.9). The dense, compact structural arrangement of the fiber distribution perpendicular to the bone surface is interlaced with a fine capillary net fed by both the PDL net and a subepithelial plexus of vessels that flows just beneath the rete peg formation. The third source of vascular supply is from larger vessels that branch from the mucosal corium just below the mucogingival junction (Fig. 3.10). The general pattern of flow is from the distal at an angle from apical to coronal through the mucogingival junction.

The arrangement of fibers in the periosteal layer of the mucosa is quite different. At the transition marked clinically by the mucogingival junction, the dense, tight attachment of fibers through the periosteum of the attached gingiva changes abruptly to a parallel layering of fibers over the periosteal layer with very little attachment to the bone (Fig. 3.11).

Between the periosteum and the lamina propria of the mucosal epithelium is a less dense submucosa of elastin, fibrillar collagen, and muscle fibers. The areolar structure of this submucosa allows for a larger vascular net in the mucosa including arterioles and large veins (Fig. 3.12).

Scattered through this matrix are active mesenchymal and inflammatory cells, which maintain and remodel the matrix; pe-

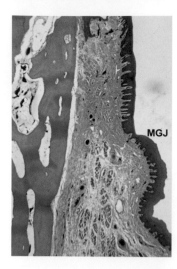

Fig. 3.13 Mucogingival junction (MGJ) transition from dense to areolar base tissue.

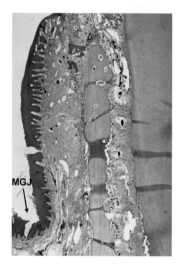

Fig. 3.14 Mucogingival junction (MGJ).

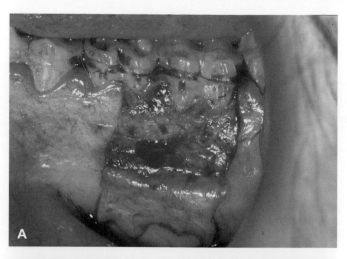

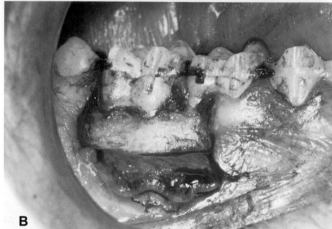

Fig. 3.15 A, Partial-thickness flap. **B,** Full-thickness flap. No vessels are exiting bone surface.

riosteal cells, which have bone-repair potential; and the cells, platelets, and soluble biomolecules contained within the vascular channels. (It is at the mucogingival junction that compaction of the gingival collagen fiber density reaches its most extreme and constricts the corium blood supply most severely) (Figs. 3.13 and 3.14).

The periosteum of the external bone surfaces receives nourishment through diffusion from connective tissue above it and seldom from true Volkman canal vessel penetrations from inside the bone outward through the cortical layers (Figs. 3.3, 3.15, and 3.16).

As previously noted, the marginal gingiva has several sources of blood flow: the PDL, the interdental, the subepithelial, and the deeper mucosal flow. The latter two sources, especially the corium or central flow, become constricted at the mucogingival junction, which is compressed like an hourglass from buccal to lingual and is further limited by the dense fiber arrangement in the gingival tissues (see Figs. 3.3 and 3.9). The degree of confinement is influenced by the biotype. In rhesus monkeys, it was observed that when the biotype was thin, there was usually only one artery (45 to 55 μm) through the mucogingival junction, while in thicker tissue, the arteries were slightly smaller (35 to 45 μm) but there were more of them (Price 1974).

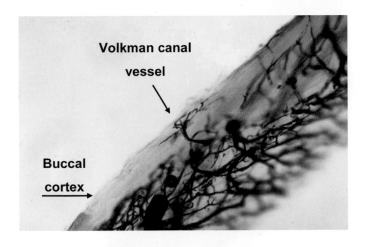

Fig. 3.16 India ink–perfused specimen.

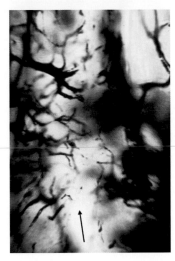

Fig. 3.17 Capillary buds at 4 days begin to cross the incision line of flap (*arrow*).

CEMENTUM

The cemental structure at the enamel level is primarily acellular with a tight adhesion to underlying dentine. While cellular cementum may persist at more apical layers, its contribution to wound healing is poorly understood. The cemental layer derives its maintenance from the surrounding PDL vessels and cells. Above the bone crest, connective tissue fibers from the attached gingiva are embedded into its surface. Below the bone crest, fibers insert into the alveolar socket wall as the principal structure of the PDL.

NORMAL EPITHELIAL STRUCTURE

Epithelial layers of the oral mucosa are connected by collagen to the underlying soft connective tissues, which in turn are connected to hard tissues such as bone and tooth structure with a variety of collagen. The epithelial seal and its reconnection to the soft connective tissues and tooth surface form the critical event in the healing process after surgical procedures. Reestablishment of this protective seal allows vascular supply, nerve, and lymphatics to permeate the underlying structures and serve as a communication network through an extracellular matrix of fibers, protein-based poly-

mers, and specific support cells, which need this protected environment.

At the tooth–enamel interface, the epithelial attachment and the gingival sulcus create an active seal that sometimes produces a flow of sulcular fluid. Near the free gingival margin, the layers thicken into a heavy, multilayered keratinized surface that continues apically on the buccal and lingual aspects of the mandible. At the mucogingival junction, this heavy gingival keratin transitions to a thinner nonkeratinized or poorly keratinized mucosal surface. On the palatal surfaces, heavy keratin is present throughout and the epithelial enclosure is punctuated by saliva and sebaceous gland openings (Fig. 3.17).

The bond of epithelial tissue to the varied underlying soft connective tissues or lamina propria is a basement membrane of Type IV collagen that may have contributions from epithelium but has collagen loops integrating from the connective tissue side. Because there are no blood vessels into the epithelial layers, the only source of its nourishment is diffusion through this basement membrane from an extensive subepithelial plexus of capillaries interconnected with the mucosal corium

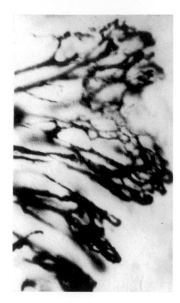

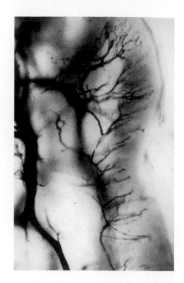

Fig. 3.18 Fourteen days: regeneration of papillary loops. At this stage, newly forming connective tissue papillas are supplied by a web of vessels.

Fig. 3.19 Twenty-one–day regeneration of papillary loops: At this stage, web has thinned out to single long arching capillaries connected to base by newly forming subpapillary plexus.

at several levels and at the alveolar socket crest with the vascular net of the PDL (Figs. 3.3, 3.17, 3.18, and 3.19).

THE WOUND-HEALING PROCESS PER SE

While the wound-healing process in periodontal surgery involves mechanisms common to other areas of the body, most notably, the skin, it has some unique features related to the presence of a tooth. Rates of activity may vary (turnover rate of alveolar bone versus basal bone) (Garant 2003), and microenvironments of local tissue architecture (attached gingiva, PDL, mucogingival junction, and so on) may influence the local microvasculature (Price 1974), but the general pattern and sequence of healing activities seem to be the same. Because vascular disruption and regeneration are central to wound-healing response, it is convenient to view the two compartments—soft tissues of gingiva/mucosa and hard tissues of tooth/bone—separately. As noted in the preceding anatomy review, while there is some interconnection, the hard tissues receive their supply from inside the bone, and the soft tissues are supplied from outside the bone.

Closure of a soft tissue wound requires epithelialization, fibroplasia, and angiogenesis, which occur simultaneously but at different rates and stages of healing. Immediately following an incision deep enough to injure the vasculature, platelets (normal range, 150,000 to 400,000/μL, produced by megakaryocytes in the bone marrow; Ganong 2001, Schmeyer 2001) are exposed to adjacent collagen and begin to adhere. This adherence activates extrusion of granules from the platelets, some of which facilitate the transformation of prothrombin to thrombin, which in turn catalyzes soluble fibrinogen to fibrin.

A fibrin net enmeshed with increasing numbers of platelets, red blood cells, circulating polymorphonucleocytes (PMNs), and macrophages contributes to an initial vascular plug or clot, which slows and stops further bleeding. This temporary or provisional matrix of cells and fibers releases a variety of chemical attractants and activators (platelet-derived growth factor [PDGF], vascular endothelial growth factor [VEGF], and transforming growth factor [TGF] ß) that stimulate the surrounding tissue layers and attract even more PMNs and macrophages from adjacent leaky venules (6 to 10 hours) (Clark 1996). The noncollagenous protein vitronectin, which is produced by the liver and circulates in the blood serum, possibly acts as a preliminary substrate for migration of these early scavenger cells.

Epithelial cells adjacent to the wound edge respond almost immediately and begin to migrate across the fibrin surface at rates estimated to be 0.5 mm/day. Within 24 hours, epithelial cells adjacent to this, formerly quiescent, begin to proliferate. Meanwhile, the PMNs in the clot begin to phagocytize bacteria, necrotic cells, and platelet debris. Resident macrophages are joined by those migrating out of the leaking vascular channels and begin to cleanse the wound of debris and broken degenerating PMNs (PMNs survive 24 to 48 hours) (Bartold 1998, Davis 2000, Garant 2003). At the same time, the macrophages release additional growth factors and cellular fibronectin, which, with fibrin, become the attachment surface for the subsequent wave of migrating cells—the fibroblasts, endothelial, and epithelial cells.

The term *fibroplasia* embodies a sequence of shifting priorities during which the fibroblast undergoes several changes in phenotypic expression. Clark in 1993 and later in 1996 described several phases: proliferation, migration, production, and transformation to myofibroblast. The proliferation phase of fibroblasts occurs in the first 2 to 3 days in the margins of the wound. These early fibroblasts are said to have vitronectin adhesion capability but not fibronectin connectivity on their membrane surfaces. By days 4 to 7, the fibroblasts switch to a migrating mode and, aided by their adhesion to fibronectin (two sources: local made by macrophages and another in circulating plasma) and fibrin, invade the space formerly occupied by the provisional matrix. As they migrate, the fibroblasts deposit collagen and matrix molecules externally (Bartold 1998, Clark 1993, Kurkinen 1980, Welsch 1990).

Angiogenesis parallels this activity with venular endothelium proliferating in place for the first few days. The cell layers thicken and the outer layer lifts off, forming a space or lumen as the endothelial intracellular cementation breaks down, enabling a migratory phase. This activity at the ends of cut vessels results in an abundance of cord-like arrays and loops that by days 4 to 5 have started to enter the clot space (see Fig. 3.17). These early activities are characterized clinically by a red, granular appearance consistent with this rapid vessel and matrix formation—the *granulation tissue.*

This granulation tissue is gradually replaced by mature fibers, matrix, and reconnected blood vessels—the *organization phase.* Extracellular fluids that had previously leaked out into the wound area during this migratory phase are resorbed, and clinical swelling begins to resolve at 5 to 6 days. At 7 days, vessels can be found to be patent but leaky, while at 14 days, the leakage has stopped (see Fig. 3.18). New circulation is mature by 21 to 28 days with gradual reduction of vessel number in favor of regular distribution and flow in the new connective tissue (Price 1974) (compare Figs. 3.18 and 3.19).

Collagens and various noncollagen molecules (hyaluron, elastin, fibronectin, and so on) are expressed into the matrix (days 4 to 10), and this in turn provides further traction and volume for migrating cells (Bartold 1998). The migrating fibroblasts now assume a fourth form (myofibroblast), which has characteristics of muscle. The combination of traction and continued migration pulls the edges of the wound inward in the phenomenon of early wound contraction, which, with continued epithelial migration, closes the wound surface (Clark 1996, Kurkinen 1980, Welsch 1990). The maturing collagen/noncollagen matrix is then in a phase where bone healing might begin (10 to 14 days). Vascular penetration in bone chambers can move at different rates in cancellous bone (0.5 mm/day) versus cortical bone (0.05 mm/day) (Rhinelander 1974a, 1974b). Osteoblasts differentiate from mesenchymal cells present within the marrow and periocytes around blood vessel walls, while osteoclasts are said to migrate from the blood vascular system (possible monocyte lineage?) (Ganong 2001, Schmaier 2003). Vascular ingrowth always precedes osteogenesis (Albrektsson 1980a, 1980b).

With the increasingly stable and maturing matrix formation, osteoblasts and osteoclasts can begin early cleanup and bone matrix deposition. Injured bone areas show osteoclast activity as early as 7 days, which persists at 14 days and is followed at 21 days by osteoblastic presence (Pfeiffer 1965).

The epithelium is mostly complete with layers by 21 to 28 days. Soft connective tissue including its vasculature continues to mature for 35 to 42 days (5 to 6 weeks) (see Figs. 3.17 through 3.19). Bone healing continues for 6 to 8 weeks, at which time a rapidly formed woven bone is present. This is gradually remodeled in a slower process, which creates mature lamellar bone. All of these events assume a stable environment with no reinjury or mobility of the site.

Intrabony healing, which is necessary after the controlled trauma of implant replacement and bone grafting, is a special situation that places increased demands on basic processes. The initial rates of activity remain the same but there are several secondary responses that need to occur for integration of either implant or graft particle. Additionally, in the case of the graft particle, it is desirable that the graft itself eventually be replaced by new bone (Branemark 1985).

The final result can be either *regeneration* (complete restitution of structure and function) or *repair* (fibrous replacement with creation of a seal).

REFERENCES

Albrektsson, T. 1980a. The healing of autogenous bone graft after varying degrees of surgical trauma. *J. Bone Joint Surg.* 62B:403–410.

Albrektsson, T. 1980b. Repair of bone graft. A vital microscopic and histological investigation in the rabbit. *Scand. J. Plast. Reconstr. Surg.* 14:1–12.

Bartold, P.M., et al. 1998. *Biology of the Periodontal Connective Tissues.* Quintessence Books, Chicago.

Branemark, P.I., et al. 1985. *Tissue-Integrated Prostheses.* Quintessence, Chicago.

Clark, R.A.F. 1993. Regulation of fibroplasia in cutaneous wound repair. *Am J. Med. Sci.* 306(1):42–48.

Clark, R.A.F. 1996. *The Molecular and Cellular Biology of Wound Repair,* 2nd ed. Kluwer Academic Publishers, Plenum Press, New York.

Folke, L.E.A., et al. 1965. Periodontal microcirculation as revealed by plastic microspheres. *J. Periosteal. Res.* 2:53–63.

Folkman, J., and M. Klagsbrun. 1987. Angiogenic factors. *Science* 23:442–448.

Ganong, W.F. 2001. *Review of Medical Physiology,* 20th ed. Lange Medical Books/McGraw-Hill, New York.

Garant, P.R. 2003. *Oral Cells and Tissues.* Quintessence, Chicago.

Ham, A.W. 1965. *Histology,* 5th ed. J.B. Lippincott, Philadelphia.

Kurkinen, M., et al. 1980. Sequential appearance of fibronectin and collagen in experimental granulation tissue. *Lab. Invest.* 43:47–51, 1980.

Pfeiffer, J.S. 1965. The growth of gingival tissue over denuded bone. *J. Periosteal.* 34:10–16, 1965.

Price, A.M. 1974. Comparison of the microvascular disruption and regeneration following full, partial, and modified partial thickness flaps in the alveolar mucosa of *Macaca mulatta*. DScD thesis, Boston University, Boston.

Rhinelander, F.W. 1974a. The normal circulation of bone and its response to surgical intervention. *J. Biomed. Mater. Res.* 8:87.

Rhinelander, F.W. 1974b. Tibial blood supply in relation to fracture healing. *Clin. Orthop.* 105:34.

Schmaier, A.H., et al. 2003. *Hematology for the Medical Student.* Lippincott Williams and Wilkins, Philadelphia.

Woodburne, A.M. 1965. *Essential of Human Anatomy,* 3rd ed. Oxford University Press, New York.

Chapter 4 The Contribution of Periodontics to Orthodontic Therapy

Donald J. Ferguson, DMD, MSD, M. Thomas Wilcko, DMD,

William M. Wilcko, DMD, MS, and M. Gabriela Marquez, DMD, MSD

Periodontally Accelerated Osteogenic Orthodontics (PAOO)

HISTORY

The innovative combination of selective alveolar periodontal decortication surgery and augmentation grafting with orthodontic treatment results in an acceleration of orthodontic treatment, enhanced stability of orthodontic results, and long-term improvement of the periodontium (Wilcko 2003). The purposes of this section are to describe the Periodontally Accelerated Osteogenic Orthodontics technique and to explain how and why this advanced periodontal surgical technique contributes to orthodontic treatment.

Decortication or *corticotomy* means simply the intentional cutting or injury of cortical bone. While the bony jaws are composed of both cortical and medullary bone in various combinations depending on site and patient demographics, the periodontal surgery of interest in contemporary selective alveolar decortication involves only surgical injury of alveolar cortical bone.

The application of corticotomy surgery to correct malocclusion was first described in 1892 by L. C. Bryan, but it was Heinrich Köle in 1959 who reintroduced alveolar corticotomy to resolve malocclusion (Köle 1959). He combined interdental alveolar corticotomy surgery with a through-and-through osteotomy apical to the teeth. Generson et al. in 1978 offered a modification of the Köle protocol and eliminated the subapical osteotomy portion of the surgery.

In 2001, Wilcko et al. described selective alveolar decortication with augmentation grafting combined with orthodontic treatment. They patented and trademarked their technique as Periodontally Accelerated Osteogenic Orthodontics (PAOO). Full-thickness labial and lingual alveolar flaps were laid adjacent to the teeth intended for movement, and selective decortication surgery was performed. Given that the surgery was done only in the area of desired tooth movement, it was the thickness of cortical bone that dictated where and how the cortical bone was injured. The depth of the decortication cuts barely penetrated into medullary bone and bleeding was promoted; care was taken not to injure any tooth or encroach on the periodontal ligament. An allograft of resorbable grafting material plus antibiotic was applied directly over the bleeding bone, and the surgical site was closed using Gore-Tex suture material. A frequently used grafting mixture was equal portions of demineralized freeze-dried bone (DFDBA) and bovine bone (Osteograf/N-300 or Bio-Oss) wetted with clindamycin phosphate (Cleocin) solution.

Wilcko et al. observed rapid orthodontics following PAOO and active treatment times of 6 to 8 months were common. They questioned Köle's precept of "bony block" movement and offered an alternative hypothesis that rapid tooth movement resulted from marked but transient decalcification-recalcification of the alveolus. Frost, an orthopedic surgeon, had described a direct correlation between degree and proximity of bone trauma and intensity of physiological healing response, which he coined Regional Acceleratory Phenomena, or RAP (Frost 1983), and the decalcification-recalcification described by Wilcko et al. (2001, 2003) was consistent with RAP.

INDICATIONS

- Increased alveolar volume and enhanced periodontium (i.e., correction of dehiscences and fenestrations)

- Accelerated treatment (i.e., 3 to 4 times more rapid active orthodontic treatment)

- Greater stability of clinical outcomes and less relapse

- Enhanced scope of malocclusion treatment (i.e., avoiding orthognathic surgery and extractions in selected cases)

- Enhancement of patient's profile when indicated

- Rapid recovery of impacted teeth (i.e., canines)

The initial decortication protocol used by the Wilcko brothers did not include augmentation alveolar grafting. Computed Tomography (CT) scans were taken on the first series of patients to compare pretreatment status with immediate post orthodontics and at least 1-year retention conditions. The CT scans of the alveolus immediately after braces were removed showed a paucity of alveolar bone in the areas where decortication surgery was performed. However, the retention images demonstrated that a minimally adequate amount of

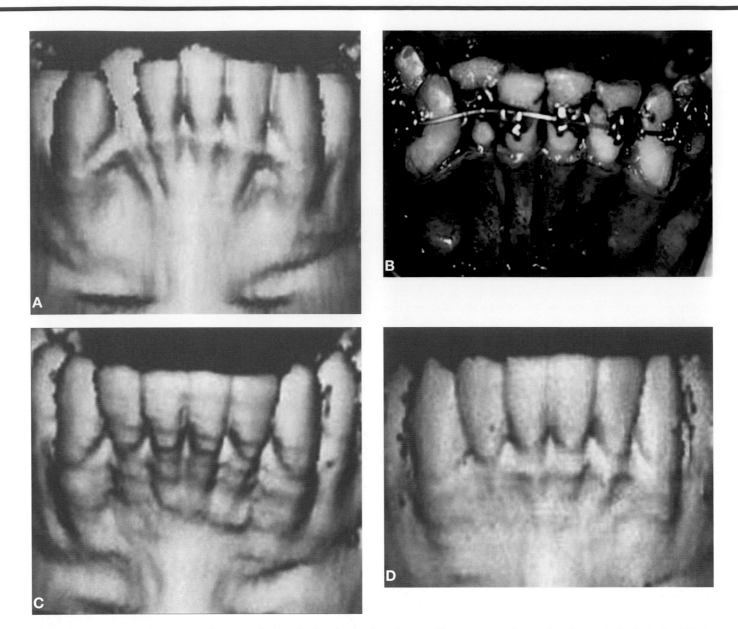

Fig. 4.1. CT and surgery images of patient treated with selective alveolar decortication without augmentation grafting demonstrating lack of calcified cortical plate at post orthodontic treatment but return of cortical plate volume by 1 year retention. **A:** CT image at pre-treatment showing root prominences; **B:** view of labial cortical bone at the time of selective alveolar decortication surgery; **C:** CT image at immediate post orthodontic treatment showing lack of calcified labial cortex; **D:** CT Image at 1 year after active orthodontic treatment showing adequate but minimal calcified labial cortex.

mineralized alveolar bone would return if the soft tissue periodontal envelope remained intact (Fig. 4.1).

Since 1996, the PAOO technique has included augmentation grafting to increase alveolar volume (Fig. 4.2). Results of research showed no change in alveolar cortical bone thickness at an average of 1.5 years following immediate post orthodontic treatment (Twaddle 2002). A recent study of attached

gingival levels in PAOO patients resulted in significantly more attached gingiva evident at least 1 year after active orthodontic treatment. Increases in attached gingiva were consistent in the lower dental arch and inconsistent in the maxillary arch (Kacewicz 2007).

An additional benefit of augmentation bone grafting is the repair of alveolar cortical bone fenestrations and dehiscences

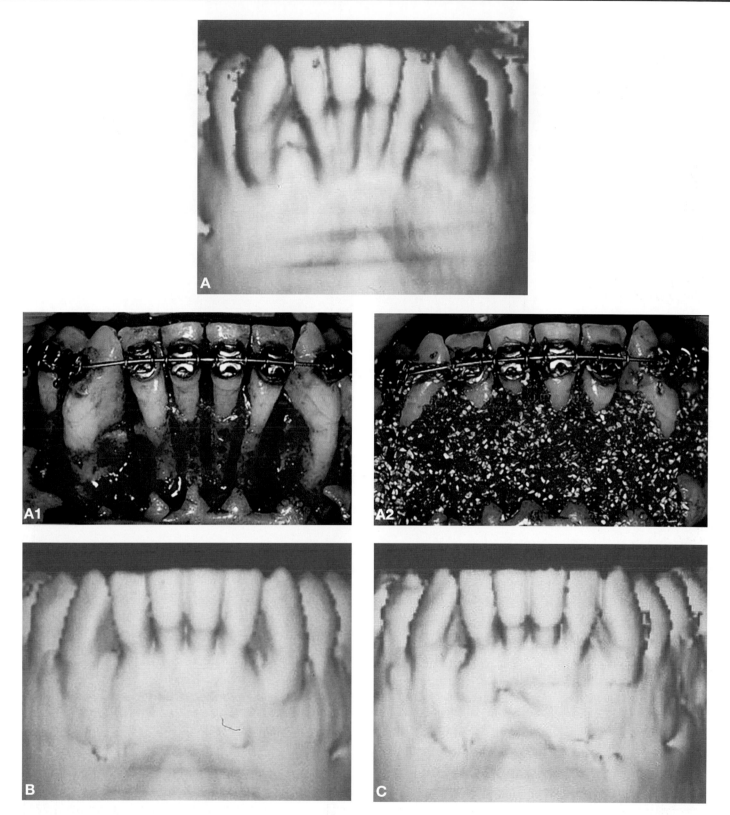

Fig. 4.2. CT and surgery images of patient treated with selective alveolar decortication and augmentation grafting demonstrating ample cortices post grafting. **A:** CT image at pre-treatment showing root prominences; **A-1:** view of labial cortical bone at the time of selective alveolar decortication surgery; **A-2:** view of surgery area after grafting; **B** & **C:** CT images at post orthodontic treatment (**B**) and 2.5 years retention (**C**) showing increased volume of labial cortical bone.

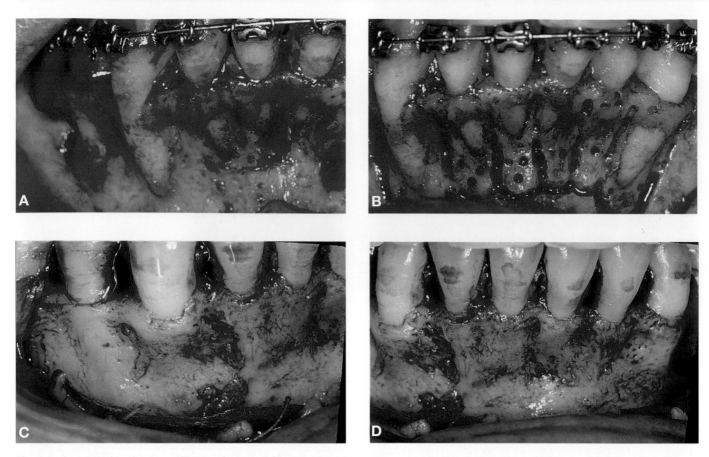

Fig. 4.3. Augmentation alveolar grafting repairs bony dehiscences and fenestrations. **A**: evidence of bony discrepancies after full thickness flap, **B**: decortication prior to grafting with dehiscences and fenestrations outlined; **C-D**: absence of dehiscences and fenestrations 7.5 years post PAOO decortication and grafting.

(Fig. 4.3). The grafting procedure is done without membranes because full-thickness flaps are used followed by primary closure in a healthy periodontium. Under these circumstances, migration of the epithelial attachment is not likely to occur, and the intact periosteum serves as a natural "membrane."

PAOO has contributed greater stability of orthodontic clinical outcomes and less relapse. Stability of orthodontic clinical outcomes was analyzed by Nazarov in 2003 using the Objective Grading System (OGS) sanctioned by the American Board of Orthodontics (ABO). While no differences were observed in nonextraction therapies at immediate post treatment between PAOO and non-PAOO groups, three of the nine OGS variables (alignment, marginal ridges, and total score) were significantly better in the PAOO group at retention. O'Hara (2005) compared nonextraction orthodontic treatment of moderate malocclusions and found no differences in the OGS alignment variables at post treatment. But at retention, alignment had improved in the PAOO group, whereas in the two non-PAOO groups, fixed and removable appliance retention, alignment had relapsed. In summary, immediate post orthodontic treatment results following nonextraction therapy are statistically the same with or without

PAOO. However, during retention, the clinical outcomes of PAOO patients improved and did not demonstrate relapse.

PAOO increases the scope of orthodontic tooth movement and the positions of the teeth after decortication and augmentation grafting are stable long-term. Sarver and Proffit (2005) offered guidelines as to the limits of central incisor tooth movement in the adult patient with orthodontic treatment alone. Ferguson et al. (2006) suggested that these limits can be expanded 2-fold to 3-fold in all dimensions except retraction following PAOO (see Fig. 4.4) and that the stability of these positions is probably due to loss of tissue memory from high turnover of the periodontium as well as increased thickness of the alveolar cortices from the augmentation grafting. Rothe et al. (2006) found that patients with thinner mandibular cortices were at increased risk for having dental relapse—hence the necessity for osseous grafting during the PAOO procedure.

Periodontics, through PAOO therapy, contributes to orthodontic treatment by reducing active orthodontic treatment time. Claims of rapid orthodontic treatment times were first validated in research by Hajji in 2000; average active ortho-

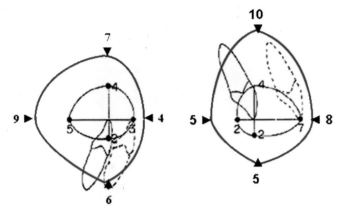

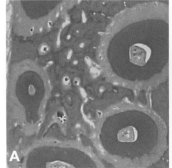
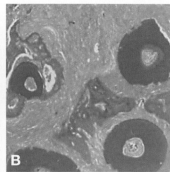
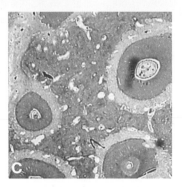

Fig. 4.4. PAOO enables a greater amount of tooth movement into stable positions. Limits of adult orthodontic tooth movement (in millimeters) into stable positions using orthodontics only is represented by the inner black-color envelope (after Proffit); limits of tooth movement for orthodontics combined with PAOO is represented by the outer red-color envelope. For example, protraction of the lower incisor into a stable position is 9mm if tooth movement is combined with PAOO compared to a 5mm limit without PAOO. Note that limits are about 2 to 3 times greater for central incisor protraction, extrusion and intrusion but not for incisor retraction. (Reprinted with permission from Bell 2006)

Fig. 4.5. Cross section of the dentoalveolus of the rat showing 4 of the 5 upper first molar roots at 3 weeks control (**A**), 3 weeks decortication (**B**), and 11 weeks decortication (**C**). Testing of histomorphometric data resulted in significantly less calcified trabecular bone volume at 3 weeks on the decortication side except for 7 weeks decortication (not shown).

dontic treatment times were 6.1 months for nonextraction PAOO and 18.7 and 26.6 for nonextraction and extraction therapies without PAOO, respectively. In 2001, Fulk compared mandibular arch decrowding in nonextraction orthodontics following PAOO and non-PAOO; active treatment times were 3.1 times more rapid (6.6 versus 20.7 months) following PAOO and post treatment outcomes were statistically the same as judged by cephalometric and study cast variables. Similar results were reported in 2003 by Skountrianos for maxillary arch decrowding, wherein active orthodontic treatment time was 3.0 times more rapid when combined with PAOO than when not combined (7.0 versus 21.2 months).

In summary, the contributions of periodontal therapy to orthodontic treatment vis-à-vis PAOO is to increase alveolar volume and enhance the periodontium, enhance the stability of orthodontic clinical outcomes (less relapse), increase the scope of malocclusion treatable without orthognathic surgery, and reduce active orthodontic treatment time over 3-fold. These benefits are realized for two reasons: (1) tissues lose memory due to high hard and soft tissue turnover induced by the periodontal decortication, and (2) augmentation bone grafting increases alveolar volume and thickness of the alveolar cortices.

BIOLOGICAL RATIONALE

The clinical technique involving selective alveolar decortication is a form of periodontal tissue engineering resulting in a transient osteopenia and high turnover adjacent to the injury site. Alveolar decortication initiates a healing response, the degree of which is directly related to the intensity and proximity of the surgical insult. In healthy tissues, bony healing is synonymous with high osseous turnover, calcium depletion from the hydroxyappatite crystal lattice, and diminished bone density but not bone matrix volume (Frost 1983). Bogoch et al. (1993) made a penetrating surgical incision into the head of the tibia in rabbits and studied the healing response adjacent to the surgical wound. They found a 5-fold increase in medullary bone turnover adjacent to the corticotomy site. Buchanan et al. (1988) documented a similar observation in alveolar bone following tooth extraction, as did Yaffe et al. (1994) after alveolar periosteal flap elevation and Verna et al. (2000) after tooth movement.

Sebaoun (2005) studied the effect of decortication without tooth movement on alveolar turnover in the rat in a split mouth design using multiple approaches. Maxillary buccal and lingual full-thickness periosteal flaps were elevated adjacent to the upper left first molar, and decortication was performed with five palatal and five buccal bur marks (0.2 mm) under sterile irrigation. The following was observed adjacent to the decortication site at 3 weeks after surgery: (1) a 2-fold increase in decalcified trabecular bone (histomorphometric analysis using hematoxylin and eosin staining; see Fig. 4.5),

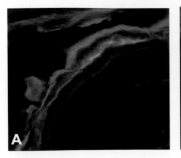

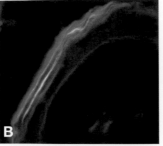

Fig. 4.6. Amount of apposition of the lamina dura is shown in cross section of the dentoalveolus of the rat at 4 weeks, the end of the first series of vital stain injections. Total width of apposition as revealed by the three stains together was statistically greater on the decortication side (**A,** 0.051mm) at 3 weeks than the control side (**B,** 0.037mm) at 3 weeks.

(2) a 1.5-fold increase in new trabecular bone formation (vital staining ad libitum), (3) a 4-fold increase is osteoclast count (osteoclast count after TRAP staining), and (4) a 2-fold increase in lamina dura apposition (vital stain injection series; see Fig. 4.6). These findings collectively indicate high tissue turnover immediately adjacent to the decortication site.

Pham-Nguyen (2006) studied the three-dimensional volume of periodontal tissues surrounding the upper first molar in the rat model following buccal and lingual selective decortication. Using micro-CT technology, a significant decrease in alveolar mineralization was evident by 7 days post decortication (Fig. 4.7).

Conceptually, increased tissue turnover (osteopenia) is a condition that favors rapid tooth movement. This tenet was demonstrated by Verna et al. (2000) using a rat model by moving teeth after pharmacologically inducing high and low bone turnover. They showed significantly greater tooth movement in the high turnover group compared with normal and low bone turnover groups. In our laboratory rat studies (Pham-Nguyen 2006, Sebaoun 2005), surgical injury to the alveolus induced a dramatic increase in tissue turnover that was expressed both spatially and temporally. The effect of alveolar decortication was localized to the area immediately adjacent to the injury. It is obvious that considerable medullary bone demineralization occurs immediately adjacent to the decortication site. Although induced osteopenia is a transient condition in the functionally normal alveolus, it was surmised that tooth movement perpetuates the decalcified condition of the trabecular bone (Fig. 4.8).

PERIODONTALLY ACCELERATED OSTEOGENIC ORTHODONTICS IN THE TREATMENT OF CROWDING

Using the PAOO technique, cases of moderate dental arch crowding are routinely completed in 4 to 6 months instead of

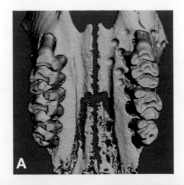

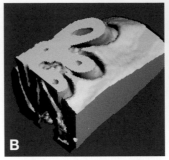

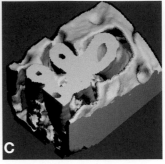

Fig. 4.7. Micro-CT analysis of osteopenia at 7 days following selective alveolar decortication showing gross specimen #602 (**A**), control side (**B**) and decortication side (**C**).On the decortication side, osteopenia was demonstrated as the bone volume (BV) to total volume (TV) ratio decreased to 45% (note the wide spaces surrounding the roots, C) compared to 57% on the control side (B). (Pham-Nguyen K, et al. 2006)

18 to 24 months of active orthodontic treatment, and the results have been shown to be remarkably stable (Figs. 4.9 and 4.10).

RAPID RECOVERY OF IMPACTED TEETH

Recovery of impacted teeth typically prolongs active orthodontic treatment time. Impacted tooth recovery combined with selective alveolar periodontal decortication surgery accelerates the recovery and reduces orthodontic treatment time. The purpose of this section is to describe an advanced periodontal surgical technique of recovering impacted cuspids that features the following: (1) complete exposure of the clinical crown, (2) clearing a path for recovery by way of alveolar ostectomy, and (3) selective alveolar decortication or intramarrow penetrations surrounding the impacted tooth root.

With the exception of the third molars, the maxillary canines are the most frequently encountered impaction, with an incidence of approximately 2% according to Ericson and Kurol (1987). The incidence of maxillary canine impaction is 3 times greater in females than in males and is often associated with missing or peg-shaped laterals (Bec et al. 1981, Peck et al. 1994). Maxillary permanent canines are impacted palatally

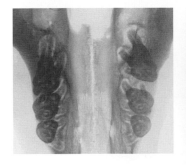
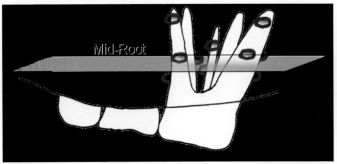
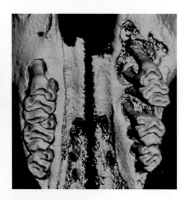
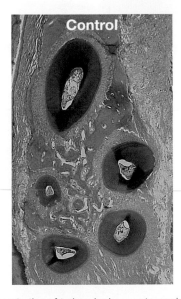
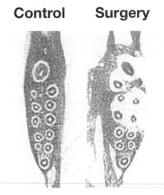
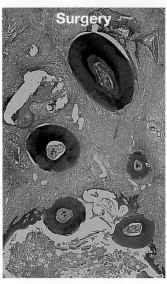

Fig. 4.8. Demonstration of trabecular bone osteopenia following decortication and 6 weeks of tooth movement in the rat. Clockwise from *upper left* image: faxitron cephalogram of animal #62 maxilla showing direction of 1st molar tooth movement; *upper center:* diagram indicating buccal (*red*) and lingual (*blue*) corticotomy cuts and histological cut through roots at mid-root level; *upper right:* gross 3D image of maxilla showing movement of 1st molar; *lower right:* H&E stain on surgery side showing lack of calcified trabecular bone surrounding the roots of the 1st molar; *lower center:* CT slice at mid-root level through 1st, 2nd and 3rd molars showing evidence of osteopenia (*white*) on surgery side compared to control side with rectangles representative of area covered in H&E stained images; *lower left:* H&E stain on control side showing ample calcified trabecular bone surrounding the roots of the 1st molar.

much more frequently than labially (85% palatal compared with 15% labial; Bass 1967, Hitchin 1956, Jacoby 1979). Rayne (1969) has pointed out that labially impacted canines are often associated with inadequate arch space. Interceptive treatment of impacted maxillary canines can often be successful in 10- to 13-year-olds depending on the degree of the impaction (Jacobs 1992). The more severely impacted maxillary canines typically require combined surgical/orthodontic treatment (Bishara 1992).

Previous authors have indicated that details of the recovery technique depend on the type of impaction. When the crown is not covered by bone and there is a broad band of keratinized gingival tissue present, Kokich and Mathews (1993), Shiloah and Kopczyk (1978), and Jarjoura et al. (2002) have suggested a surgical window (gingivectomy) to expose the

shallow impaction. In situations where there is only a narrow zone of gingival attachment and a relatively shallow labial or mid-alveolar bony impaction, an open technique consisting of an apically repositioned flap is more suitable according to Wong-Lee and Wong (1985) and Vanarsdall and Corn (1977). When the bony impaction is deep in the vestibule, mid-alveolar, or impacted palatally, Vermette et al. (1965), McDonald and Yap (1986), and Smukler et al. (1987) have suggested erupting the canine through the gingiva following primary surgical flap closure.

RECOVERY OF LABIALLY IMPACTED CANINES

Recovery of labially impacted maxillary canines is illustrated in the treatment of a girl aged 14 years 4 months using selec-

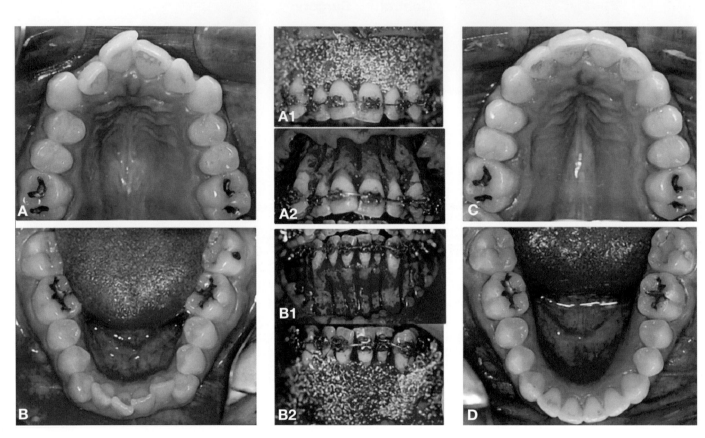

Fig. 4.9. Adult female patient with moderate upper and lower dental arch malocclusion (**A,B**) treated by PAOO (**A-1, A-2, B-1, B-2**) showing immediate post treatment outcome after 7 months of active orthodontic therapy (**C,D**).

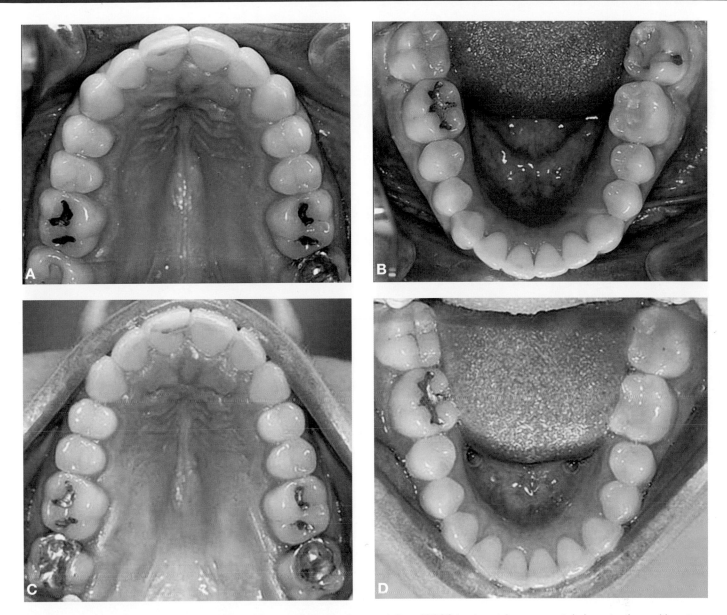

Fig. 4.10. Retention outcome at 2 years (**A,B**) and 9 years (**C,D**) after the completion of PAOO treatment. Improvement during retention and long term stability are likely due to high tissue turnover induced by decortication and increase in cortical bone thickness.

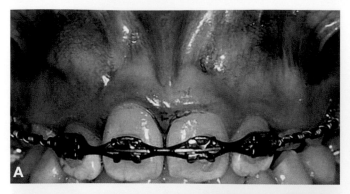

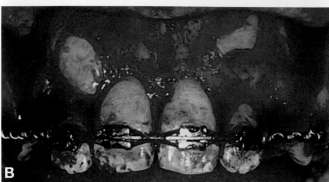

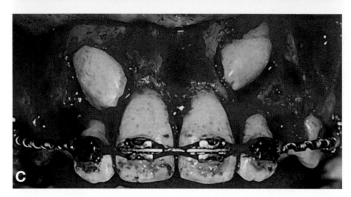

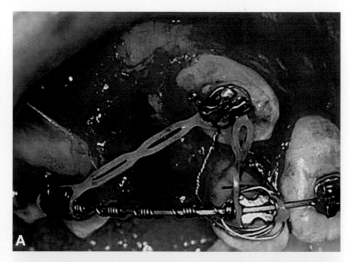

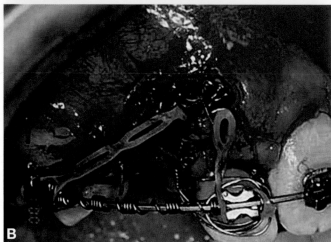

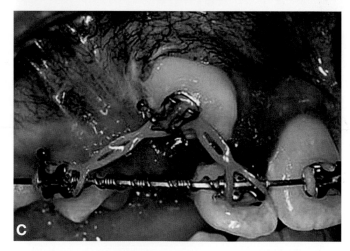

Fig. 4.11. Labially impacted maxillary canines showing pre-surgery (**A**), partial exposure of canine crowns after full-thickness flap (**B**), and bone removal to expose canine crowns completely, intramarrow penetrations, and creation of a path by removing facial cortical plates of extraction socket (**C**).

Fig. 4.12. Treatment for labially impacted maxillary canines showing views of different cases at the time of surgery (**A, D, G, B, E, H**) and at 10 weeks post surgery (**C, F, I**). An orthodontic bracket was placed in an optimal position on the exposed right canine (**A**) but on the lingual surface of the crown on the left canine (**G**). At the time of soft tissue closure, a vertical incision was made in the flap allowing exposure of the right canine bracket (**B**) but not the left canine (**H**) before suturing the flap to the original position (**E**). The canines were beginning to move rapidly by 10 weeks after the canine recovery surgery (**C, F, I**).

tive decortication technique (Figs. 4.11, 4.12, and 4.13). A full-thickness labial flap, using a sulcular incision with vertical releasing incisions mesial to the first premolars, was reflected to reveal upper cuspid crowns labial to the upper permanent lateral incisors. No lingual flap was reflected. The upper primary canines were extracted, and the soft tissue follicle and thin layer of bone surrounding cuspid crowns were removed. A path (trough) was cleared for the forced eruptions by removing the facial cortical plate between the cuspid crowns and extraction sockets including the facial plates over the sockets. In addition, numerous intramarrow penetrations were made to stimulate alveolar bone turnover and to induce

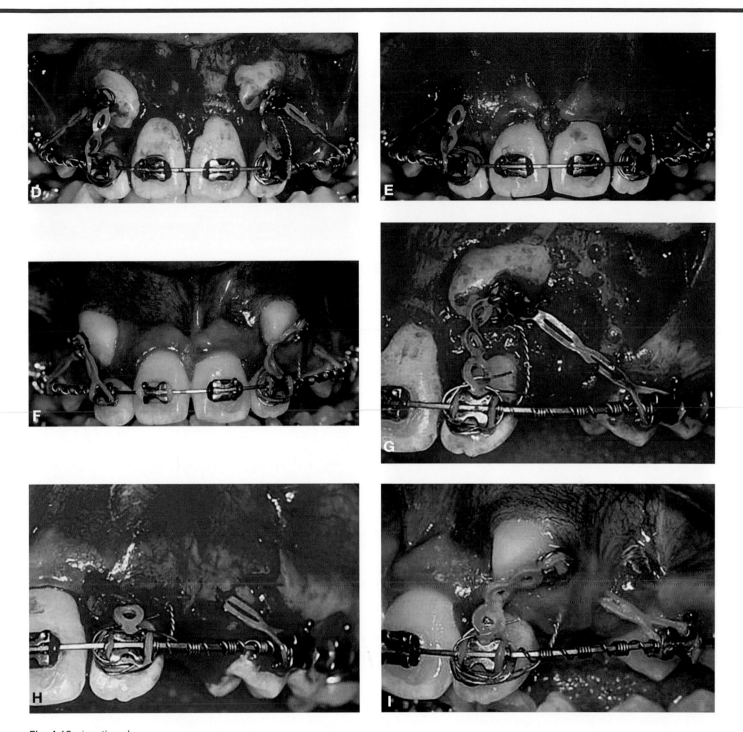

Fig. 4.12. (continued)

RAP or osteopenia. At least 1.5 mm of bone was left undisturbed mesial to the first premolars and distal to lateral incisors. An orthodontic bracket was placed in an optimal position of the upper right permanent canine, but the upper left permanent canine was rotated, which necessitated placing the bracket on the lingual surface. On the right side, the bracket was exposed with a vertical incision in line with the bracket, and then suturing the flap back into the original position. The upper left canine was covered by the flap and sutured back in its original position. Because the upper left canine was covered by the flap, a backup ligature wire was also used. In this case, a resorbable Vicryl suture was used.

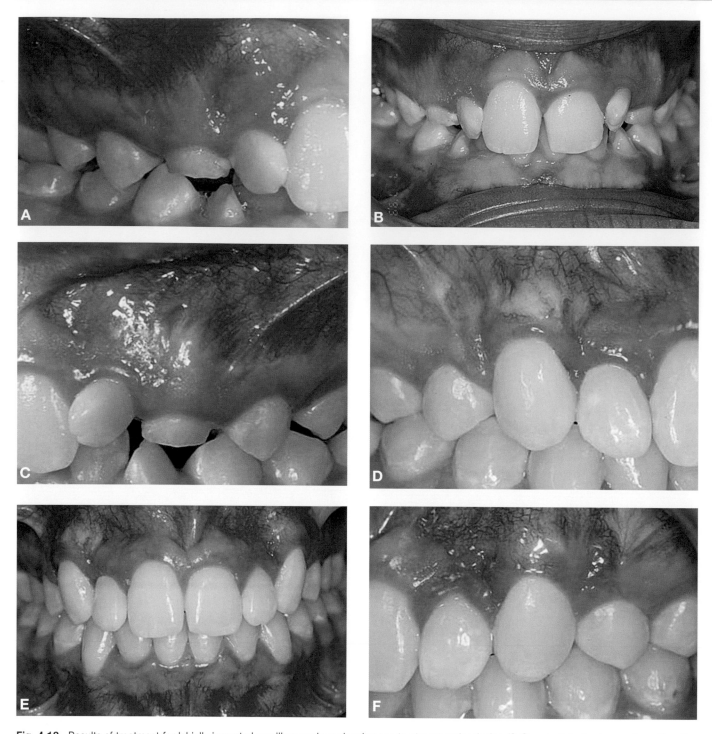

Fig. 4.13. Results of treatment for labially impacted maxillary canines showing pre-treatment malocclusion (**A-C**) and clinical outcome 4 months after removal of orthodontic appliances (**D-F**). Active treatment time to recover the canines was 5 months and 2 weeks.

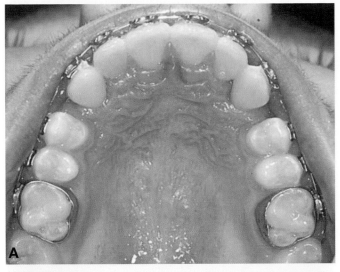

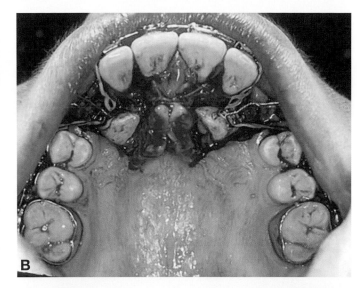

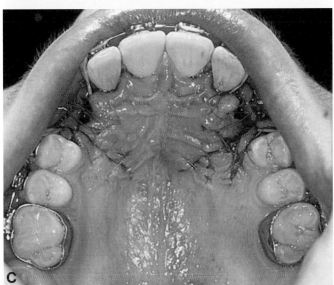

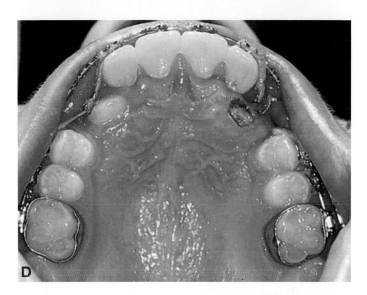

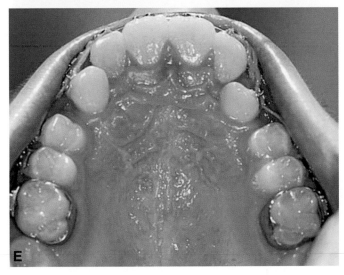

Fig. 4.14. Treatment for deep palatally impacted maxillary canines showing pre-treatment malocclusion (**A**), canine exposure, bracketing and elastic traction (**B**), flap repositioning and suturing (**C**), 3 months post surgery (**D**), and complete canine recovery (**E**). Active treatment time to recover the canines was 6 months and 0 weeks.

RECOVERY OF DEEP PALATALLY IMPACTED CANINES

Selective decortication is especially helpful in the recovery of maxillary permanent canines that are deeply impacted on the palatal side and require a considerable amount of movement through alveolar medullary bone as illustrated with the treatment of a boy aged 14 years 6 months (Figs. 4.14 and 4.15). Decortication injury stimulates an osteopenic response that reduces the mineral content of spongiosa, thereby reducing the resistance to impacted canine movement.

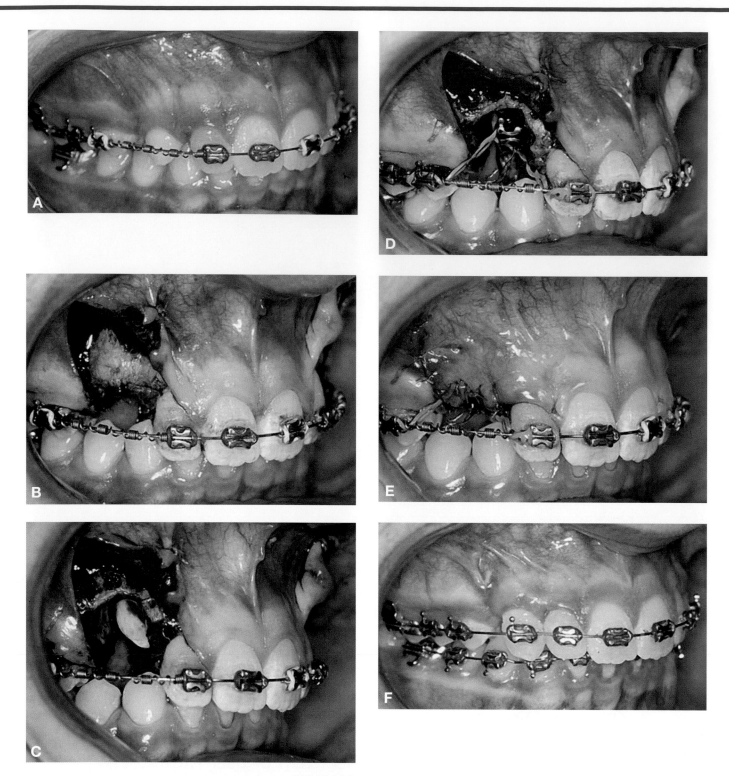

Fig. 4.15. Treatment for deep palatally impacted maxillary canine showing pretreatment malocclusion (**A**) and radiograph (**H**), flap with vertical releasing incision showing labial cortical plate (**B**), ostectomy removal of labial cortical and medullary bone to clear a movement path and expose canine crown, and labial intramarrow penetrations (**C**), bracket placement and application of elastic traction (**D**), immediate postsurgical flap suturing (**E**) and radiograph (**F**) with radiograph (**I**), and 9 days after orthodontic appliance removal (**G**) with radiograph (**K**). Active treatment time to recover the canine was 6 months 0 weeks.

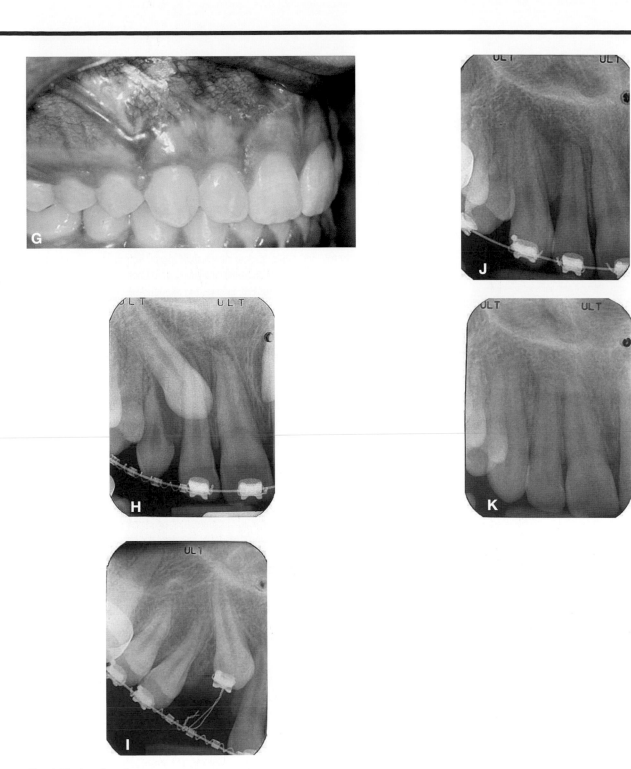

Fig. 4.15. (*continued*)

Both facial and lingual full-thickness flaps are used with distal vertical releasing incisions for access to deep palatally impacted canines. Preference is given to placement of orthodontic brackets into an optimal positioned on the labial surface of the canine crown for control and efficiency. When direct access to the labial surface and optimal bracket placement is not possible, the surface of choice for bracket placement is the distolabial surface of impacted canines. An ostectomy is required between the first premolar and the lateral incisor to gain access to the appropriate impacted canine surface. The ostectomy not only permits optimal bracket placement but also creates a space for the elastic chain from the bracket on the impacted canine to the brackets on the adjacent teeth already well positioned in the dental arch. Moreover, bone needs to be removed when crowns are exposed because the follicle surrounding the enamel is eliminated and bone resorption secondary to follicular activity is lost. The ostectomy should eliminate all bone in the movement path of the crown during impacted canine recovery, but it is important to leave about 1.5 mm of bone on the proximal surfaces of the adjacent teeth. Intramarrow penetrations are also performed, especially in the bone that lies between the impacted tooth and its eventual position in the dental arch. Intramarrow penetrations over the root prominence of the impacted tooth facing in the direction of movement stimulate medullary osteopenia and reduce tooth movement resistance. After the bracket has been placed, a ligature wire is secured to the bracket of the impacted tooth as backup in the event the elastic chain was to break. A bracket with a post or power arm pointing apically is preferred to reduce the likelihood of the chain elastic slipping off the bracket. The full-thickness flaps are returned to their original positioning and sutured. In the case demonstrating recovery of deep palatally impacted canines (Figs. 4.14 and 4.15), nonresorbable 5-0 green braided polyester suture material was used, but the type of suture material used is usually not relevant. Suture removal, when necessary, is recommended anytime after 1 week of postoperative healing.

PERIODONTAL SURGICAL PROCEDURES FOR ORTHODONTIC ACCESS, AESTHETICS, AND STABILITY

Excessive gingival attachment serves no useful purpose before, during, or after orthodontic treatment. There are several reasons for excessive gingival attachment. Gingival excess can result from systemic medications that produce undesirable side effects of gingival hyperplasia such as dilantin, nifedipine, and amlodipine or gingival swelling such as cyclosporine; thick, fibrotic gingival overgrowth can produce tooth movement and/or malocclusion. Excessive gingival attachment can result from familial hereditary gingival hyperplasia or, more commonly, by delayed passive eruption of teeth (Fig. 4.16).

Surgical removal of gingiva is called *gingivectomy,* and *gingivoplasty* refers to recontouring the gingival architecture

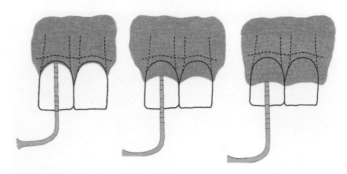

Fig. 4.16. Delayed passive eruption of teeth can lead to excessive gingival attachment: normal attachment (*left*), moderate excess attachment (*center*), and severe excess attachment (*right*). Note that the tip of the periodontal probe rests at the gingival crest demonstrating that clinical crown length deceases as gingiva excess increases.

and/or changing the gingival shape. These simple periodontal surgical procedures can contribute meaningfully to orthodontic access, aesthetics, and treatment outcome stability. The fundamental reasons for gingivoplasty procedures are to provide more optimal clinical crown appearances or access and to change gingival shape. According to Sarver (2004), exposure of the clinical crowns that contribute most to the aesthetic smile, the maxillary central incisors, should be approximately 80% width compared with height. Moreover, the gingival architecture for the anterior teeth should have certain characteristics. The gingival shape of the mandibular incisors and the maxillary laterals should exhibit a symmetrical half-oval or half-circular shape, and the maxillary centrals and canines should exhibit a gingival shape that is more elliptical. Thus, the gingival zenith (the most apical point of the gingival tissue) should be located distal to the longitudinal axis of the maxillary centrals and canines, and the gingival zenith of the maxillary laterals and mandibular incisors should coincide with their longitudinal axis (Fig. 4.17).

Excessive gingival attachment often makes optimal orthodontic bracket placement difficult. When the patient is ready for orthodontic treatment with fixed appliances but access to the clinical crown precludes optimal bracket position placement, a gingivoplasty procedure can be used to establish a more favorable crown-to-crestal height relationship by removal of excess gingiva. This is a frequent finding in young patients ready for orthodontic treatment in the late mixed or early permanent dentition (Fig. 4.18).

Removal of excessive gingival tissues is useful during the course of orthodontic treatment to facilitate good oral hygiene and to help in the consolidation of the dental arch

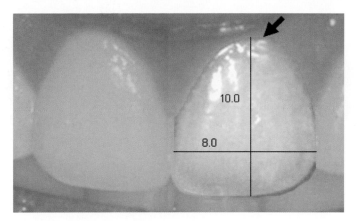

Fig. 4.17. Optimal maxillary incisor exposure for esthetics is 1.0 to 0.8 crown height-to-width ratio and ideally, gingival zenith or most apical point of the gingival tissue is distal to longitudinal crown axis. (After: Sarver MS, AJODO, 126:749-753, 2004.)

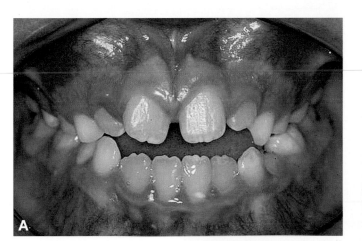

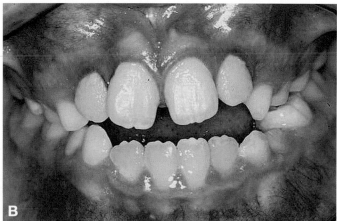

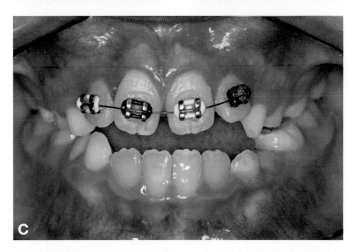

Fig. 4.18. Increasing access to upper incisor clinical crowns for bracketing on an 11 year old orthodontic patient: pre-treatment (**A**), 15 days post gingivoplasty (**B**), and post incisor bracketing (**C**).

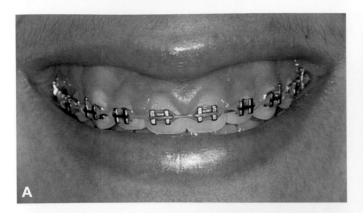

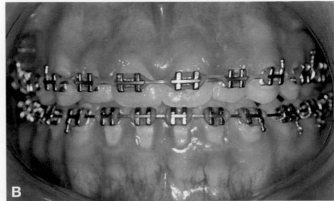

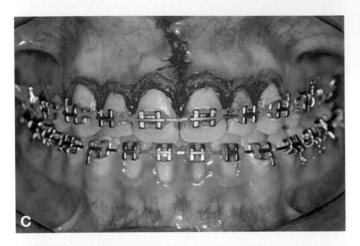

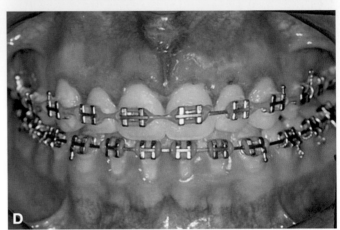

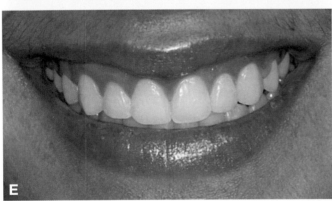

Fig. 4.19. Removal of excessive upper anterior gingiva was accomplished during the course of active orthodontic treatment in a 15 year old patient: pre-gingivoplasty (**A,B**), gingivoplasty and frenectomy (**C**), and 7 days after the gingivoplasty (**D**) and post orthodontic treatment (**E**).

spacing and orthodontic detailing and finishing. Moreover, gingivoplasty at least 2 weeks before removal of fixed orthodontic appliances allows sufficient gingival healing to enable the fabrication of an overlay, Essix type of orthodontic retainer that is well adapted to the gingival contours (Fig. 4.19).

Post orthodontic gingivoplasty can contribute to both smile aesthetics and stability of treatment outcomes (Fig. 4.20). The supracrestal gingival fibers have been identified as con-

tributing to orthodontic relapse, especially rotation relapse, and consequently the procedure called *supracrestal fibrotomy* has been recommended (Edwards 1988). Others have suggested that orthodontic treatment outcome stability is more likely due to an increase in the elasticity of the whole compressed gingival tissue (Redlich et al. 1996). In either case, gingivoplasty influences the turnover and adaptation of both supracrestal and compressed gingival tissues, thereby reducing orthodontic treatment outcome instability.

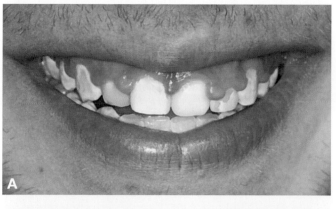

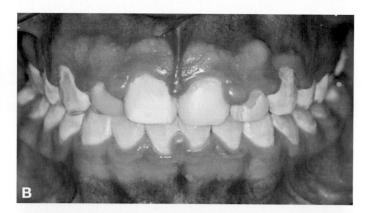

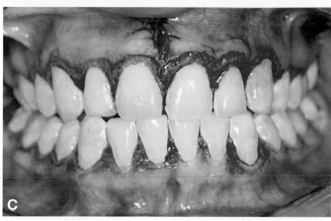

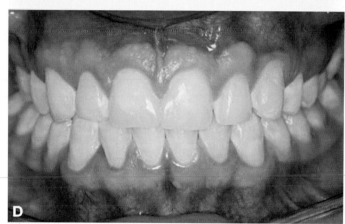

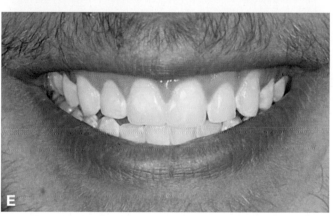

Fig. 4.20. Effect of recontouring gingival architecture to improve the esthetics an d stability of orthodontic treatment outcome in a 18 year old male patient; immediate post orthodontics (**A,B**), immediate post gingivectomy (**C**) and 4 months post gingivectomy (**D,E**).

REFERENCES

Anholm, J.M., D.A. Crites, R. Hoff, and W.E. Rathbun, 1986. Corticotomy facilitated orthodontics. *Calif. Dental Assoc. J.* 14:7–11.

Bass, T.B. 1967. Observations on the misplaced upper canine tooth. *Dental Pract. Dental Rec.* 18:25–30.

Bec, A., P. Smith, and R. Behar. 1981. The incidence of anomalous maxillary lateral incisors in relation to palatally displaced cuspids. *Angle Orthod.* 51:24–29.

Bishara, S.E. 1992. Impacted maxillary canines: a review. *Am. J. Orthod. Dentofac. Orthop.* 101:159–171.

Bogoch, E., N. Gschwend, B. Rahn, E. Moran, and S. Perren. 1993. Healing of cancellous bone osteotomy in rabbits, part I: regulation of bone volume and the RAP in normal bone. *J. Orthop. Res.* 11:285–291.

Buchanan, M., H.S. Sandhu, and C. Anderson. 1988. Changes in bone mineralization pattern: a response to local stimulus in maxilla and mandible of dogs. *Histol. Histopathol.* 3:331–336.

Edwards, J.G. 1988. A long-term prospective evaluation of the circumferential supracrestal fiberotomy in alleviating orthodontic relapse. *Am. J. Orthod. Dentofac. Orthop.* 93:380–387.

Ericson, S., and J. Kurol. 1987. Radiographic examination of ectopically erupting maxillary canines. *Am. J. Orthod. Dentofac. Orthop.* 91:483–492.

Ferguson, D.J., W.M. Wilcko, and M.T. Wilcko. 2006. Selective alveolar decortication for rapid surgical-orthodontic resolution of skeletal malocclusion. In W.E. Bell and C. Guerrero, editors. *Distraction Osteogenesis of the Facial Skeleton.* BC Decker, Hamilton, Ontario, Canada.

Frost, H.A. 1983. The regional acceleratory phenomena: a review. *Henry Ford Hosp. Med. J.* 31:3–9.

Fulk, L.A. 2001. Lower arch decrowding comparing corticotomy-facilitated, midline distraction and conventional orthodontic techniques. Master's degree thesis in orthodontics, Saint Louis University.

Gantes, B., E. Rathburn, and M. Anholm. 1990. Effects on the periodontium following corticotomy-facilitated orthodontics. *J. Periodontol.* 61:234–238.

Generson, R.M., J.M. Porter, A. Zell, and G.T. Stratigos. 1978. Combined surgical and orthodontic management of anterior open bite using corticotomy. *J. Oral Surg.* 36:216–219.

Hajji, S.S. 2000. The influence of accelerated osteogenic response on mandibular decrowding. Master's degree thesis in orthodontics, Saint Louis University.

Hitchin, A.D. 1956. The impacted maxillary canine. *Br. Dental J.* 100:1–14.

Jacobs, S.G. 1992. Reducing the incidence of palatally impacted maxillary canines: a useful preventative interceptive orthodontic procedure: case report. *Austral. Dental J.* 37: 6–11.

Jacoby, H. 1979. The "Batista spring" system for impacted teeth. *Am. J. Orthod.* 75:43–51.

Jarjoura, K., P. Krespo, and J.B. Fine. 2002. Maxillary canine impactions: orthodontic and surgical management. *Comp. Cont. Educ. Dent.* 23:23–38.

Kokich, V., and D.P. Mathews. 1993. Surgical and orthodontic management of impacted teeth. *Dent. Clin. North Am.* 37:181–204.

Köle, H. 1959. Surgical operations on the alveolar ridge to correct occlusal abnormalities. *Oral Surg. Oral Med. Oral Pathol.* 12:515–529.

Machado, I.M., D.J. Ferguson, W.M. Wilcko, and M.T. Wilcko. 2002. Reabsorcion radicular despues del tratamiento ortodoncico con o sin corticotomia alveolar. *Rev. Venezuelana Orthod.* 19:647–653.

McDonald, F., and W.L. Yap. 1986. Surgical exposure and application of direct traction of unerupted teeth. *Am. J. Orthod.* 89: 331–340.

Nazarov, A.D. 2003. Improved retention following corticotomy using BO Objective Grading System. Master's degree thesis in orthodontics, Saint Louis University.

O'Hara, P. 2005. Orthodontic treatment and retention outcomes with and without PAOO and fixed retainers. Master's thesis in orthodontics, Boston University.

Peck, S., and M. Kataja. 1994. The palatally displaced canine as a dental anomaly of genetic origin. *Angle Orthod.* 64:249–256.

Pham-Nguyen, K. 2006. Micro-CT analysis of osteopenia following selective alveolar decortication and tooth movement. Master's degree thesis in orthodontics, Boston University.

Rayne, J. 1969. The unerupted maxillary canine. *Dental Pract. Dental Rec.* 19:194–204.

Redlich, M., E. Rahamim, A. Gaft, and S. Shoshan. 1996. The response of supra-alveolar gingival collagen to orthodontic rotation movements in dogs. *Am. J. Orthod. Dentofac. Orthop.* 110:247–255.

Rothe, L.E. 2006. Trabecular and cortical bone as risk factors for orthodontic relapse. *Am. J. Orthod. Dentofac. Orthop.* 129:316.

Rothe, L.E., A.M. Bollen, R.M. Little, S.W. Herring, J.B. Chaison, C.S.K. Chen, and L.G. Hollender. 2006. Trabecular and cortical bone as risk factors for orthodontic relapse. *Am. J. Orthod. Dentofac. Orthop.* 130:476–484.

Sarver, D.M., and W.R. Proffit. 2005. Special considerations in diagnosis and treatment planning. In T.M. Graber, R.L. Vanarsdall, and K.W.L. Vig, editors. *Orthodontics: Current Principles and Techniques.* Elsevier, St. Louis, p. 15.

Sarver, D.M. 2004. Principles of cosmetic dentistry in orthodontics: part 1. Shape and proportionality of anterior teeth. *Am. J. Orthod. Dentofac. Orthop.* 126:749–753.

Sebaoun, J.D. 2005. Trabecular bone modeling and RAP following selective alveolar decortication. Master's degree thesis in orthodontics, Boston University.

Shiloah, J., and R. Kopczyk. 1978. Mucogingival considerations in surgical exposure of maxillary canines: report of case. *ASDC J. Dent. Child.* 45: 79–81.

Skountrianos, H.S. 2003. Maxillary arch decrowding and stability with and without corticotomy-facilitated orthodontics. Master's degree thesis in Orthodontics, Saint Louis University.

Smukler, H., G. Castellucci, and H.M. Goldman. 1987. Surgical management of palatally impacted cuspids. *Comp. Cont. Educ. Dent.* 8:10–77.

Suya, H. 1991. Corticotomy in orthodontics. In E. Hösl and A. Baldauf, editors. *Mechanical and Biological Basics in Orthodontic Therapy.* Hüthig, Heidelberg, pp. 207–226.

Twaddle, B.A., D.J., Ferguson, W.M., Wilcko, M.T., Wilcko, and C.-Y. Lin. 2002. Dento-alveolar bone density changes following accelerated orthodontics. *J. Dental Res.* 80:301.

Vanarsdall, R.L., and H. Corn. 1977. Soft tissue management of labially positioned unerupted teeth. *Am. J. Orthod.* 72:53–66.

Vermette, M.E., V.G. Kokich, and D.B. Kennedy. 1995. Uncovering labially impacted teeth: apically positioned flap and closed eruption technique, *Angle Orthod.* 65:23–32.

Verna, C., M. Dalstra, and B. Melsen. 2000. The rate and type of orthodontic tooth movement is influenced by bone turnover in the rat model. *Eur. J. Orthod.* 22:343–352.

Wilcko, W.M., D.J. Ferguson, J.E. Bouquot, and M.T. Wilcko. 2003. Rapid orthodontic decrowding with alveolar augmentation: case report. *World J. Orthod.* 4:197–205.

Wilcko, W.M., M.T. Wilcko, J.E. Bouquot, and D.J. Ferguson. 2001. Rapid orthodontics with alveolar reshaping: two case reports of decrowding. *Int. J. Periodont. Restor. Dent.* 21:9–19.

Wong-Lee, T.H., and F.C. Wong. 1985. Maintain an ideal tooth-gingival relationship when exposing and aligning an impacted tooth. *Br. J. Orthod.* 12:189–192.

Yaffe, A., N. Fine, I. Alt, and I. Binderman. 1994. Regional accelerated phenomena in the mandible following mucoperiosteal flap surgery. *J. Periodontol.* 65:79–83.

Miniscrew Implants for Orthodontic Anchorage

HISTORY

Implants for use as orthodontic anchorage devices have recently become very popular because most are easy to place and remove and inexpensive and can be directly or indirectly loaded with biomechanical forces immediately after placement. Unlike the osseointegrated implants used for prosthetic restorations, implants for orthodontic anchorage rely on mechanical retention and depend on the thickness of cortical bone for stability (Huja 2005). This screw-in type of implant is known by many names such as temporary anchorage devise (TAD), mini-implant, microscrew, or miniscrew.

Implants for orthodontic anchorage were first described in the literature in 1945 by Gainsforth and Higley and were used to retract the canine tooth in the dog model. In 1983, Creekmore and Eklund reported placement of a screw device in the anterior nasal spine area for use in the intrusion of upper permanent incisors in the treatment of adult deep bite malocclusion. Kanomi in 1997 provided detailed description of loading microimplants less than 1.0 mm in diameter following 3 months of osseous integration. Since 2000, the dental literature has been inundated with articles describing new designs and the use of immediate-load implants as anchorage devices for the treatment of malocclusion. In general, they have proved successful for intrusion and extrusion, protraction, and retraction of individual teeth as well as groups of teeth.

Miniscrew implants are the smallest among all fixed implants; they are the most versatile and adaptable for clinical use and are categorized as either non–bracket-head or bracket-head. The most commonly used implant for orthodontic anchorage is self-drilling with a nonbracket head. These self-drilling and self-tapping (a different cutting point for self-drilling) miniscrews have emerged during the past 6 years as the most popular and frequently used type of orthodontic anchorage implant, and this type of miniscrew will be the focus of this chapter.

Desirable features of a miniscrew include the screw threads, soft tissue sleeve or transmucosal collar, platform, and head (Fig. 4.21). The screw thread portion interfaces with cortical bone; the transmucosal collar interfaces with the soft tissues of the periosteum, either keratinized or nonkeratinized; the

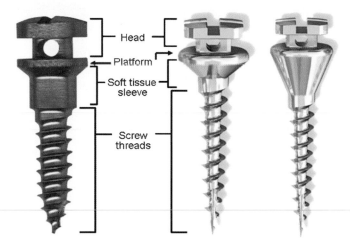

Fig. 4.21. Desirable features of self-drilling miniscrews include the screw threads, soft tissue sleeve or transmucosal collar, platform and head. *Left*: Self-drilling miniscrew with non-bracket head (Courtesy of KLS Corporation). *Middle* and *Right*: Self-drilling, self-tapping Spider Screw K1 short transmucosal collar (*middle*) and long neck (*right*) with bracket like head (Courtesy of Ortho Technology, Inc. exclusive distributor of Spider Screw products for HDC Italy.)

platform or soft tissue stop protects the soft tissue from the attachments that connect the miniscrew to the orthodontic appliance and also decreases the likelihood of tissue overgrowth around the screw head; and the head provides the means (often a round hole) for connecting the miniscrew to the orthodontic appliance as well as the screwdriver slots for applying self-drilling and self-tapping pressure.

INDICATIONS

- When "absolute" orthodontic anchorage is needed
- Adequate cortical bone thickness and quality
- Healthy soft and hard tissues of the periodontium

Miniscrews are now considered a reliable anchorage device for orthodontic treatment. Since Food and Drug Administration approval in 1999, these devices have broadened the scope of treatment possibilities not only in orthodontics but in periodontics and prosthodontics as well. Without the use of

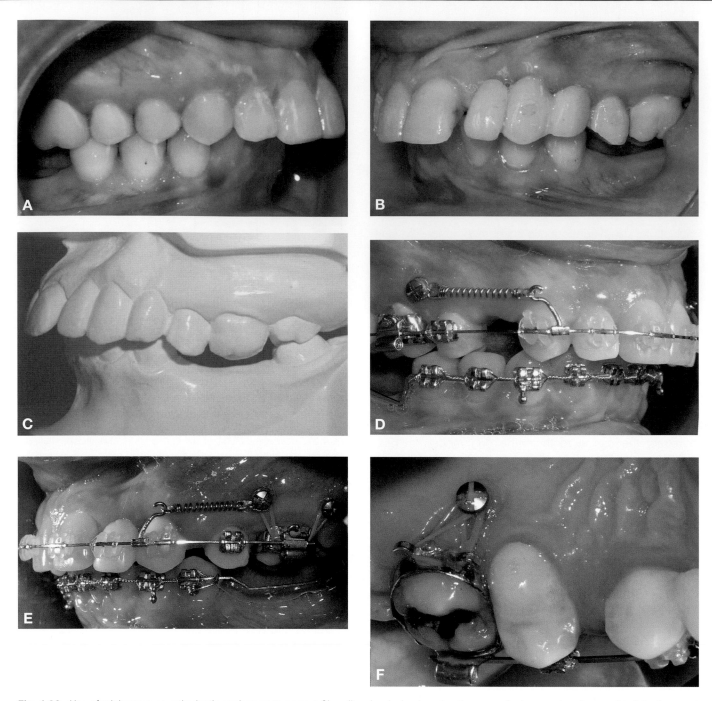

Fig. 4.22. Use of miniscrews as orthodontic anchorage to correct Class II malocclusion by retracting upper incisors and canines and to intrude upper left first molar: pre-treatment (**A-C**), during treatment (**D-F**) and completed treatment (**G-I**). Note placement of miniscrew at junction of attached gingiva and mucosa during treatment and use of palatal implant to assist with molar intrusion. Also note the interocclusal space created by intrusion of the upper left premolar and molar.

implants, forces are generated using other structures as anchorage such as teeth in order to produce desired orthodontic tooth movement. Teeth used as anchorage will inevitably respond with some movement because the anchor teeth are surrounded by a periodontal ligament (PDL), and the PDL is sensitive and responsive to changes in the environment. Miniscrews implanted into cortical bone are stable and do not

respond like teeth because the screw threads interface directly with cortical bone as there is no mechanism like the PDL that enables movement of the implant.

Miniscrew implants are most appropriate when there is a need for "absolute" anchorage. They should be inserted into keratinized gingiva if possible and loaded immediately

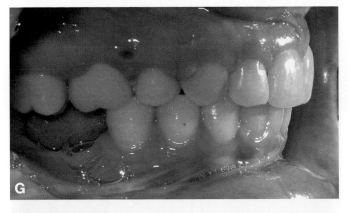

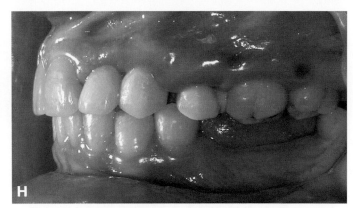

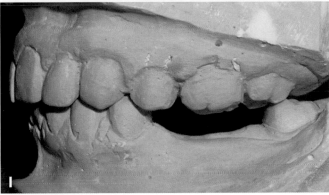

Fig. 4.22. (*continued*)

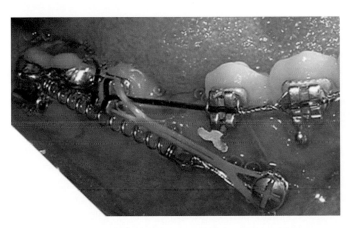

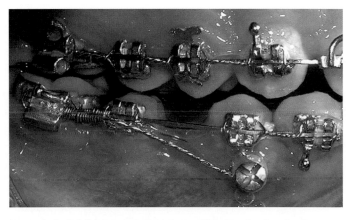

Fig. 4.23. Two uses of miniscrew as orthodontic anchorage to protract posterior teeth: *Left:* Miniscrew used to secure NiTi closed coil spring for molar protraction and elastic chain for premolar protraction. *Right:* Open coil spring placed mesial to molar allows protraction of the premolar only; steel ligature tie from miniscrew to molar prevents distal molar movement. Note the less desirable placement of the miniscrew below mucogingival junction (*left*) and more desirable placement of the miniscrew at junction of attached gingiva and mucosa (*right*).

(Melsen and Costa 2000) or within the first 2 weeks of healing (Liou et al. 2004). These devices are effective as anchorage for moving teeth in three spatial planes such as retracting the upper incisors and canines in the treatment of Class II malocclusion following first premolar extraction or intrusion of molars (Fig. 4.22) or protracting posterior teeth to close space (Fig. 4.23).

Miniscrew stability depends on cortical bone thickness because spongy bone contributes virtually nothing to implant stability (Melsen 2005). Alveolar bone is composed of compact (cortical) and spongy (trabecular or medullary) bone. Medullary bone is a highly adaptable tissue, and it responds quickly to changes in the environment with modeling or surface change, whereas cortical bone responds

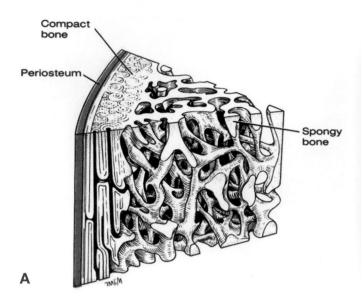

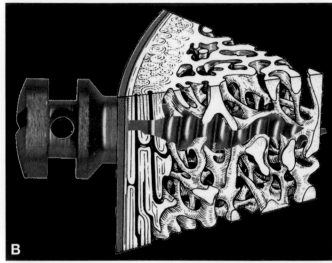

Fig. 4.24. Diagrams illustrating the differences in cortical and spongy bone response to a miniscrew. **A:** Compact or cortical bone undergoes remodeling, a coupled sequence of activation then resorption then formation (A-R-F), whereas spongy bone undergoes modeling which is activation followed by either resorption or formation (A-R or A-F). **B:** Miniscrew implanted into slow turnover cortical bone and rapid reacting spongy bone; miniscrew stability comes from cortical bone.

slowly to stimuli with remodeling or internal change. Bone modeling is an uncoupled activity of activation (A) followed by formation (F) or resorption (R). Because an activation can lead to either resorption (A-R) or formation (A-F), spongy bone very quickly adapts to any stimuli or change in environment. In contrast, compact bone undergoes bone remodeling which is a coupled sequence of activation (A) followed by resorption (R) followed by formation (F) or A-R-F sequence. The A-R-F sequence is otherwise known as the process of secondary osteon formation: physiological activation (a stimulus) followed by bone resorption (cutting cone) followed by bone formation (filling cone). Remodeling (A-R-F) is a slow process that assures structural integrity of the host skeleton (Roberts et al. 2004). The principal reason for miniscrew implant stability is attributed to the slow bony turnover response of cortical bone (Fig. 4.24).

Miniscrew thread lengths vary from 4 mm to 12 mm with longer thread lengths recommended for bicortical retention (Freudenthaler et al. 2001). In most circumstances, miniscrew thread length need not exceed the width of monocortical thickness. A miniscrew thread length of 6 mm should be adequate and a 4-mm thread length is optimal under most circumstances because monocortical alveolar bone thickness ranges between 2 and 3.5 mm on the facial or lingual mandible in the areas of the first and second molars (Masumoto et al. 2001) and 2 and 7 mm in the palate

(Bernhart et al. 2000, King et al. 2006). The soft tissue sleeve width should be at least 2.5 mm, as this is approximately the average thickness of keratinized soft tissue of the periodontium (Costa et al. 2005). Some manufacturers provide short and long transmucosal collars to accommodate variations of soft tissue thickness.

Some situations contraindicate use of miniscrews, according to Park et al. (2003). Miniscrews are contraindicated in the presence of active infection such as untreated periodontal disease and when there is inadequate bone quantity such as in severe alveolar bone loss. When bone quality is compromised, as in untreated osteoporosis or a history of systemic drug use to counteract calcium depletion, miniscrews may be contraindicated. Miniscrews should not be used when there is a limitation in blood supply, when patients are incapable of following home care instructions, and during the mixed dentition if there is risk of permanently damaging tooth buds. The small size of the miniscrews for the most part precludes any permanent tissue damage (Kanomi 1997); root perforation is unlikely and any minor root damage will heal uneventfully (Mah and Bergstrand 2005). No litigation concerning miniscrew use has yet been reported; however, case selection should be carefully considered. An informed consent should be presented to the patient, fully explaining the benefits and risks (including pain, bleeding, inflammation, implant fracture and implant mobility, and/or failure) of using miniscrews.

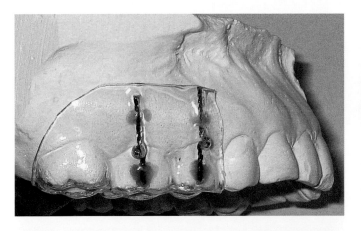
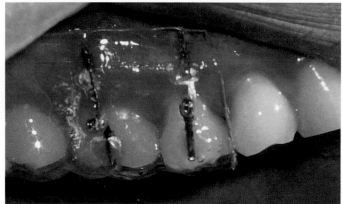
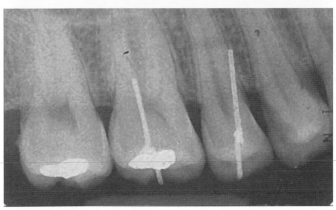
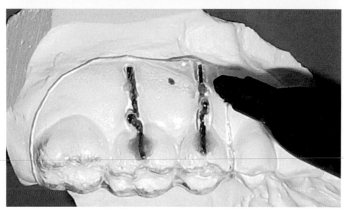

Fig. 4.25. Example of an implant guide or "jig" fabricated to assist in the placement of a miniscrew implant: Vacuum-type retainer fabricated on study cast incorporating wire adapted approximating the long axis of 1st molar and 2nd premolar (*top left*); transfer of guide to patient's mouth (*top right*); radiographic image of patient with guide seated (*bottom left*); and transfer of guide back to study cast to mark position of miniscrew placement after measuring distance between wires on the radiograph (*bottom right*).

ARMAMENTARIUM

- Self-drilling or self-tapping miniscrews

- Profound topical anesthetic or an injectable anesthetic

- Manual screwdriver or slow-speed handpiece with appropriate screwdriver attachment

Technique

The overall soft and hard tissue periodontal condition of the patient should be thoroughly evaluated and healthy before miniscrew placement and application of biomechanical forces. Self-drilling miniscrews are easy to place and can be implanted under local soft tissue anesthesia or with the use of a topical anesthetic alone (Graham 2006). A profound topical anesthetic is preferred because anesthetizing the teeth alters the patient's perception of increased resistance to screwdriver pressure (suggesting contact with a root) and a change in sensitivity from pressure to sharp pain. If resistance is encountered during placement, the miniscrew should be backed away and redirected or removed completely and placed elsewhere. Melsen (2005) suggests at least 1 month of healing if there is a desire to place a miniscrew at the identical location of a previous miniscrew. When a miniscrew needs to be relocated immediately, she suggests at least a 5-mm distance from the initial implant site. Vital structures such as major blood vessels, nerves, maxillary sinus, and tooth roots need to be avoided during implant placement. The use of a guide or "jig" and a vertical bitewing as a reference point to determine the location of insertion can be useful in miniscrew placement (Figs. 4.25 and 4.26).

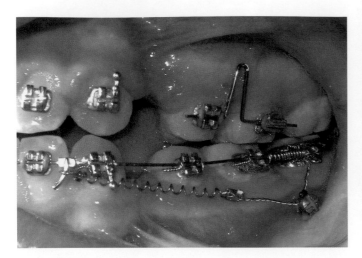
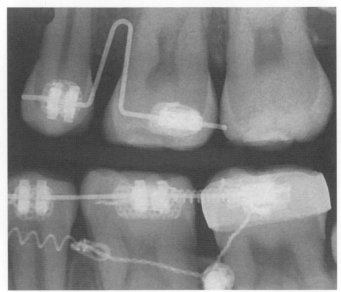

Fig. 4.26. Example of a guide fabricated with fixed orthodontic appliances in place. An arch wire segment placed in the brackets of the upper second premolar and first molar with loop extended toward vestibule (*left*). A bitewing radiograph shows the position of wire loop relative to the roots of the two teeth (*right*). The clinician will place the miniscrew mesio-apical to the height of the wire loop.

Optimal placement of the miniscrew is into attached or keratinized gingiva or at the junction of attached gingiva and mucosa (Fig. 4.27). Keratinized gingiva is abundant on the hard palate but usually limited on the buccal or labial alveolus. An apically directed insertion is suggested when the band of attached gingiva is thin or the attached gingiva level is coronal to the mid-root.

Depending on design, some miniscrews require drilling a pilot hole using a dental handpiece before insertion. Self-drilling and self-tapping miniscrews are placed without the assistance of a preliminary tap-hole and require only a screwdriver to turn the screw. Miniscrews can be inserted using a slow-speed handpiece attachment, but the use of a hand-manipulated screwdriver is more common. Whenever a manual screwdriver is used, irrigation is not necessary; however, a slow insertion speed should be used to minimize the heat generated in the bone. The type of equipment needed to insert the implant device depends on the screw diameter, screw design (cylindrical versus conical), location (palate versus buccal-labial), and recipient's bone density.

Where the miniscrew is to be inserted should be determined based on the biomechanical requirements and type of mechanics as well as the root proximity. The location of miniscrew placement between the permanent second premolar and first molar at the level between mid-root to apex is frequently used in orthodontics because this location typically provides adequate cortical bone thickness (Masumoto 2001) and is both convenient and strategic as a biomechanical anchorage site. In general, the hard palate provides ample cor-

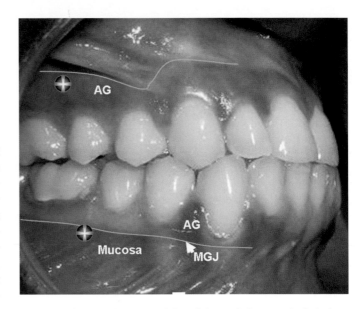

Fig. 4.27. Optimal placement of the miniscrew is into attached gingiva (AG) or at the junction of the mucosa and attached gingiva (MGJ). The miniscrew should be directed apically during insertion if the band of attached gingiva is thin.

tical bone thickness, and all soft tissue is keratinized. Alveolar cortical bone is typically thinner in the maxilla than in the mandible and thinner in females than in males, and the canine fossa regions can be particularly thin and problematic for miniscrew retention (Costa et al. 2005).

Clinical success of the miniscrew is determined by implant stability as long as it is being used as an anchorage device. No randomized clinical trials have yet been published but many case reports describe miniscrew failure rates (screw loss or mobility) ranging from 3% to 50% (Cheng et al. 2003, Deguchi et al. 2003, Melsen 2005B, Miyawaki et al. 2003). The stability depends on mechanical retention at the interfaces of the cortical bone and the screw threads; physical factors that influence stability are screw diameter, thickness of cortical bone, and placement orientation (Miyawaki et al. 2003). There is a direct relationship between miniscrew diameter and stability but an inverse relationship between miniscrew diameter and ease of placement with screw thread diameters over 2.5 mm. Self-drilling miniscrews with diameters greater than 2.5 mm become difficult to place and screws less than 1.0 mm in diameter are at risk for implant fracture, increased instability and/or complete failure (loss). The optimal range of self-drilling miniscrew diameter is between 1.5 and 2.0 mm. Placement of a miniscrew perpendicular to cortical bone surface is acceptable when cortices are at least 2 mm thick, but when cortical bone is thinner, changing the orientation of the screw and inserting in a more apical direction allows greater screw thread to cortical bone contact and greater stability. Optimally, the miniscrew should be placed into keratinized attached gingival or at least at the boundary between attached gingival and unbound mucosal tissue. While some implant systems advocate placement in mucosa to favor distance and/or vector of force between the miniscrew and the target teeth, inflammation and soft tissue overgrowth are often problems. In those cases where miniscrew placement in mucosa cannot be avoided, a soft tissue punch prior to insertion is highly recommended to prevent the loose tissue from engaging the threads of the screw. A postinsertion radiograph should be taken to confirm appropriate location of the miniscrew, and a 1-week follow-up visit whenever possible is recommended to check for pain, peri-implantation soft tissue inflammation, and stability. After treatment has been completed, removal of the miniscrew does not require anesthesia.

COMPLICATIONS

- Miniscrew mobility
- Peri-implantation inflammation
- Soft tissue injury
- Root damage
- Root resorption/bone loss
- Sinus perforation
- Implant fracture

Complications are less likely to occur with self-drilling or self-tapping miniscrews than with immediate load orthodontic anchorage systems that require soft tissue incisions or surgical flaps during placement. Complications that may arise during self-drilling and/or self-tapping miniscrew placement and use include the following.

Miniscrew Mobility

Instability occurs when the interface between cortical bone and miniscrew is not sufficient to provide adequate support for the implant. The most common scenarios are when cortical bone is too thin or when there is sufficient thickness of the alveolar cortex, but soft tissue thickness is excessive, the miniscrew is too short, and screw threads do not sufficiently implant into bone. Failing to load the miniscrew within 2 weeks of placement promotes epithelial proliferation in the interface of the bone and miniscrew and is another reason for excessive implant mobility. Miniscrews often become loose in patients with compromised bone quality resulting from some systemic bone conditions or the therapeutic effects of osteoporosis/osteopenia treatment. The miniscrew should be adequate if it is stable enough to withstand the loading forces; however, if mobility is excessive, then the miniscrew should be removed.

Peri-implantation Inflammation

Placing miniscrews into alveolar mucosa introduces the risk of soft tissue inflammation and overgrowth with the miniscrew head buried and out of reach. The risk of soft tissue inflammation can be reduced by prescribing and using clorohexidine rinses for 7 days starting the day of the miniscrew insertion into alveolar mucosa. When miniscrews are used, home care instruction should be carefully explained to the patient and monitored throughout the treatment, especially when miniscrews are placed into nonkeratinized periodontal soft tissues.

Soft Tissue Injury

Soft tissue injury may result during placement of a miniscrew into alveolar mucosa if a soft tissue punch is not used before insertion because the loose mucosa easily engages the threads of the screw. Attachments from the fixed orthodontic appliance to the head of the screw can injure soft tissue; this problem can be minimized by using screws designed with soft tissue stops or platforms.

Root Damage

Minor root damage usually heals with no consequence (Mah and Bergstrand 2005), especially if the damaged PDL area does not exceed 2 mm (Andreasen and Kristerson 1981). If the damage is greater than 2 mm, ankylosis and/or external/internal root resorption may result. In these situations develop, close radiographic monitoring is recommended.

Root Resorption/Bone Loss

Root resorption can be the result of excessive force, especially during intrusion. Park et al. (2003) used between 200g

and 300g force to intrude posterior teeth without noticeable root resorption or vitality problems. Melsen et al. (1988) reported that following tooth intrusion, periodontal tissue was recovered by new attachment only when good hygiene was enforced. Intrusion under unhealthy conditions can precipitate bone loss; therefore, a 3-month recall regimen is recommended for all patients undergoing intrusion movement.

Sinus Perforation

Sinus perforation can be easily avoided by close inspection of the patient's radiographs. Pneumatization of the sinus can increase the likelihood of perforation. If the communication does not exceed 2 mm, no further action needs to be taken.

Implant Fracture

The greater the miniscrew diameter, the less likely it is that the implant will fracture or break. Miniscrews with diameters exceeding 1.5 mm are easy to place, and the likelihood of screw breakage is minimal. A broken miniscrew should be removed unless the retrieval effort will result in an excessive amount of tissue removal.

Complications in the placement and use of self-drilling and self-tapping miniscrews are infrequent. As with other forms of therapy, complications are minimized when miniscrews are placed, used, and monitored with careful and continuous attention to the patient's physical anatomy, health, and well-being.

REFERENCES

Andreasen, J.O., and Kristerson, L. 1981. The effect of limited drying or removal of the periodontal ligament: Periodontal healing after replantation of mature permanent incisors in monkeys. *Acta Odontol. Scand.* 29:1–13.

Bernhart, T., A. Völlgruber, A. Gahleitner, O. Dortbudak, and R. Haas. 2000. Alternative to the median region of the palate for placement of an orthodontic implant. *Clin. Oral Implant Res.* 11:595–601.

Cheng, H.C., E. Yen, L.S. Chen, and S.Y. Lee. 2003. The analysis of failure using Orthoanchor K1 mini-implant system as orthodontic anchorage. *J. Dent. Res.* 82(Spec Issue B):B-214:1624.

Costa, A., G. Pasta, and G. Bergamaschi. 2005. Intraoral hard and soft tissue depths for temporary anchorage devices. *Semin. Orthod.* 11:10–15.

Creekmore, T.D., and M.K. Eklund. 1983. The possibility of skeletal anchorage. *J. Clin. Orthod.* 17:266–269.

Deguchi, T., T. Takano-Yamamoto, R. Kanomi, J.K. Hartsfield, Jr., W.E. Roberts, and L.P. Garetto. 2003. The use of small titanium screws for orthodontic anchorage. *J. Dent. Res.* 82:377–381.

Freudenthaler, J.W., R. Haas, and H.P. Bantleon. 2001. Bicortical titanium screws for critical orthodontic anchorage in the mandible: a preliminary report on clinical applications. *Clin. Oral Implants Res.* 12:358–363.

Gainsforth, B.L., and L.B. Higley. 1945. A study of orthodontic anchorage possibilities in basal bone. *Am. J. Orthod. Oral Surg.* 31:406–416.

Graham, J.W. 2006. Profound, needle-free anesthesia in orthodontics. *J. Clin. Orthod.* 40:723–724.

Huja, S.S. 2005. Biologic parameters that determine success of screws used in orthodontics to supplement anchorage. In J.J. McNamara, editor. *Implants in Orthodontics.* Ann Arbor, MI.

Kanomi, R. 1997. Mini-implant for orthodontic anchorage. *J. Clin. Orthod.* 31:763–767.

King, K.S., E.W. Lam, M.G. Faulkner, G. Heo, and P.W. Major. 2006. Predictive factors of vertical bone depth in the paramedian palate of adolescents. *Angle Orthod.* 76:743–749.

Liou, E.J., B.C. Pai, and J.C. Lin. 2004. Do miniscrews remain stationary under orthodontic forces? *Am. J. Orthod. Dentofac. Orthop.* 126:42–47.

Mah, J., and F. Bergstrand. 2005. Temporary anchorage devices: a status report. *J. Clin. Orthod.* 39:132–136.

Masumoto, T., I. Hayashi, A. Kawamura, K. Tanaka, and K. Kasai. 2001. Relationship among facial type, buccolingual molar inclination, and cortical bone thickness on the mandible. *Eur. J. Orthod.* 23:15–23.

Melsen, B. 2005. Intraoral extradental anchorage. In J.A. McNamara, editor. *Implants in Orthodontics.* Ann Arbor, MI.

Melsen, B., N. Agerbaek, J. Eriksen, and S. Terp. 1988. New attachment through periodontal treatment and orthodontic intrusion. *Am. J. Orthod. Dentofac. Orthop.* 94:104–116.

Melsen, B., and A. Costa. 2000. Immediate loading of implants used for orthodontic anchorage. *Clin. Orthod. Res.* 3:23–28.

Melsen, B., and C. Verna. 2005. Miniscrew implants: the Aarhus Anchorage System. *Semin. Orthod.* 11:24–31.

Miyawaki, S., I. Koyama, M. Inoue, K. Mishima, T. Sugahara, and T. Takano-Yamamoto. 2003. Factors associated with the stability of titanium screws placed in the posterior region for orthodontic anchorage. *Am. J. Orthod. Dentofac. Orthop.* 124:373–378.

Park, Y.C., S.Y. Lee, D.H. Kim, and S.H. Jee. 2003. Intrusion of posterior teeth using mini-screw implants. *Am. J. Orthod. Dentofac. Orthop.* 123:690–694.

Roberts, W.E., A. Huja, and J.A. Roberts. 2004. Bone modeling: biomechanics, molecular mechanics and clinical perspectives. *Semin. Orthod.* 10:123–161.

Chapter 5 The Contribution of Periodontics to Endodontic Therapy: The Surgical Management of Periradicular Periodontitis

Mani Moulazadeh, DMD

HISTORY AND EVOLUTION

Over the past century, surgical endodontics has been performed for treatment and conservation of teeth with persistent post endodontic treatment infections.

In 1964, with the formation of the American Association of Endodontists and establishment of endodontics as a dental specialty, surgical endodontics began to take a new face. Early on, much emphasis was placed on development of a root-end filling material that would provide a hermetic seal.

While magnification and the use of a microscope for operations date back to the early 1920s, it was not until 1984 when it was used in conjunction with an apical surgery (Reuben and Apotheker 1984). With the addition of the surgical operating microscope (SOM) to the armamentarium, the technique and outcome for apical surgeries became more conservative and predictable. After all, one cannot treat what one cannot see, and with the magnification of up to ×30 and illumination of up to ×12 with the dental overhead light, the SOM can reveal details previously unseen to the surgeon. The use of the SOM has become the standard of care in all endodontic procedures, and since 1998, all postgraduate programs in endodontics in the United States are required to train their residents to perform procedures under the SOM. As a result, instruments have been either newly designed or modified by scaling them down to a fraction of their original size to be used with the SOM. Ultrasonic tips and micromirrors were developed in the mid-1980s for the purpose of retropreparation and inspection under the SOM. Along with the introduction of new root-end filling material such as ProRoot mineral trioxide aggregate (MTA; Dentsply Tulsa Dental, Tulsa, OK, USA), the art of endodontic surgery has shifted toward endodontic microsurgery and has reached new heights in its levels of precision, predictability, and success.

Today, microsurgical endodontics is considered to be the standard of care. With the advent of SOM, microinstruments, superior retrofilling material, and more advanced hard and soft tissue management techniques, procedures are more conservative and outcomes have become more successful. Smaller osteotomy windows are made to conserve cortical bone. Root resection with shorter or no bevel angles, previously impossible due to lack of ultrasonic tips, are now feasible and conserve more root structure in order to preserve a more favorable crown-to-root ratio. The SOM allows for locating and treating isthmuses and extra portals of exit along the root's long axis, ensuring a proper orientation and depth for the placement of a root-end filling. It also enables the surgeon to check for marginal integrity of the apical seal once it is placed. This prevents leaving avenues for leakage, which will prevent the formation of an impermeable seal and may ultimately result in treatment failure. Rubinstein and Kim (1999, 2002) reported the short-term (1 year) and long-term (5 to 7 years) success rates for endodontic microsurgery to be 96.8% and 91.5%, respectively. These results are rather impressive considering that about 60% of the surgeries were performed on premolars or molars.

TOOTH CONSERVATION VERSUS IMPLANTS

With the recent implant paradigm shift in dentistry, some clinicians have made claims as to suggest the placement of immediate load implants is a more logical treatment over treatment of the teeth via endodontics (Ruskin et al. 2005). As clinicians, we must not be easily affected or swept away by advertisements or reading one such article. Rather, our decisions for selecting treatment plans, modalities, and techniques should be made on an evidence-based approach to dentistry and its specialties. Many have attempted to overplay the success of dental implants over nonsurgical and surgical endodontic therapy. However, in a systematic review of the literature (M.K. Iqbal and S. Kim, unpublished data) there were no significant differences between root canal therapy success rates and implants. In fact, comparing the "success" rates of endodontics and implants is sometimes beyond the scope of comparing apples and oranges.

Endodontically treated teeth are evaluated for success on the basis of clinical and radiographic criteria. An endodontically treated tooth that is asymptomatic while in function and displays no periapical radiolucency is classified as a successful treatment. Implants are often evaluated for their "success" based on their survival rate. This disparity in the evaluation criteria between endodontics and implants immediately changes the "level ground" for comparison. In addition, implant studies often exclude patients who have underlying systemic diseases such as diabetes, smokers, and patients with poor oral hygiene. In certain studies peri-implantitis was not regarded as a criterion for implant failure. Also, at least presently, most implants in these studies are being placed by trained specialist.

Meanwhile, the success of endodontic therapy as evaluated by studies did not abide to the same strict patient exclusion criteria as did the implant studies. Persistent radiographic demineralization was considered to be a sign of failure. Last, the success rate of endodontic therapy as reported by such studies as the Toronto Study is based on treatments performed by dental students, general dentists, and endodontists. In 1999, American Dental Association reported that only 25% of all endodontic cases were being performed by endodontists (ADA Report 1999).

It is clear that implants have changed the face of dentistry and the way we treatment plan restoring edentulous spaces. They are a great adjunct when treatment is planned properly and when bone quality and aesthetics allow for their placement. Implants are clearly not an alternative for periodontally sound and endodontically treatable (nonsurgical or surgical) teeth. Retaining our patients' healthy natural dentition should be our main priority as health care providers.

TREATMENT OF FAILED ROOT CANAL THERAPY

When the initial root canal therapy has resulted in a negative outcome, two revisions are possible:

- Nonsurgical retreatment aimed to eliminate bacteria from the canal

- Surgical retreatment aimed to encapsulate bacteria inside the canal

The decision as to which approach to take should be based on the level of evidence and other criteria such as the dentist's training and experience, availability of the necessary armamentarium, and the patient's decision based on informed consent.

Historically, nonsurgical retreatment has enjoyed a higher success rate than the surgical approach. Studies also support that in the event of a surgical approach, prior nonsurgical retreatment will increase the chance of a positive outcome (Zuolo 2000). Therefore, unless nonsurgical retreatment is not feasible due to physical, anatomical, time, or financial hardships, surgical endodontics should not be considered as the treatment of choice.

RATIONALE FOR ENDODONTIC SURGERY

Periapical surgery is performed to eradicate persistent infection/inflammation associated with teeth with previously negative post-treatment outcome from either initial endodontic therapy or retreatment. With advancement in microsurgical endodontics, surgery should not be labeled as a last option, but it should be performed when either initial endodontic treatment or retreatment is not possible or feasibly cannot secure a better outcome. Factors such as inability to properly access the root canal system in order to adequately clean, shape, and obtain an apical seal may warrant surgery as the treatment of choice. The ability of the clinician to properly diagnose which case is suitable for surgery is as important as his or her clinical skills. It was Dr. Irving J. Naidorf who said, "A good surgeon knows how to cut, and an excellent surgeon knows when to cut" (Kim 2002).

INDICATIONS FOR ENDODONTIC SURGERY

Anatomical Challenges

In certain cases, the tooth anatomy renders itself unwilling to proper debridement and obturation, leaving a portion of canal untreated by nonsurgical methods. Teeth with canal blockages due to severe calcification or with severe radicular curvatures fall under such category.

Also, in a few cases when endodontic therapy is performed at a clinically acceptable level, symptoms may continue to persist when the apex of the root may be fenestrating through the facial cortical plate of bone. In these cases, a small surgical procedure to recontour the root end and align it within its bony housing may solve the problem.

Iatrogenic Factors

Previous endodontic "misadventures" account for the need for surgery in cases with persistent symptoms. These include but are not limited to canal blockages, ledges, perforations, separated instruments or posts, underfilled canals, and canals with dental material extruding beyond the biologically tolerant buffer zone around the anatomical apex (Figs. 5.1 through 5.3).

In most of these cases, proper canal debridement is compromised as is the ability to properly obturate the canal and obtain a proper apical seal.

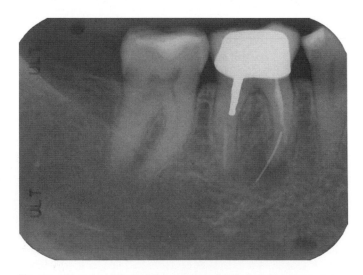

Fig. 5.1. Persistent inflammation associated with the mesial root of a mandibular molar with a separated instrument.

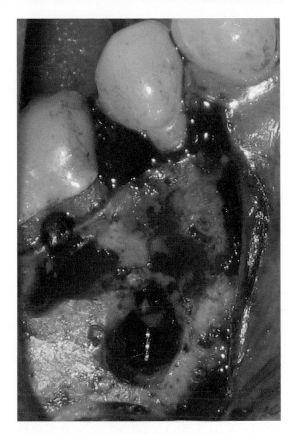

Fig. 5.2. Surgery reveals a hand file extending 3 to 4 mm beyond the root tip.

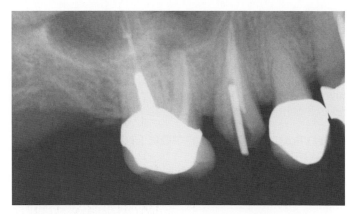

Fig. 5.4. Persistent inflammation and symptoms associated with the mesial root of a maxillary molar due to the missed MB-2 canal.

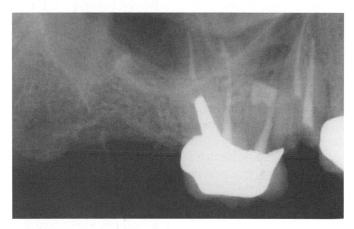

Fig. 5.5. Apicoectomy performed in conjunction with finding and obturation of the additional canal and the isthmus between MB-1 and MB-2 canals.

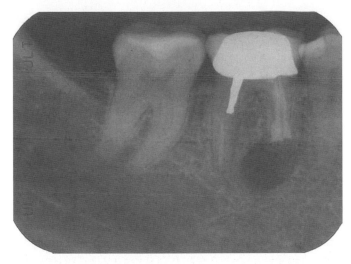

Fig. 5.3. Instrument recovery, root resection, and retrograde obturation with MTA.

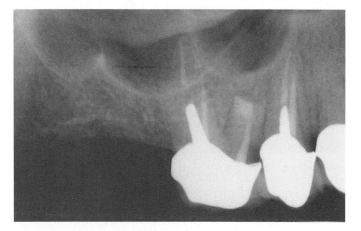

Fig. 5.6. A 4-year follow-up shows complete healing.

Relentless Inflammation

Previously missed and untreated canals, bifurcations, fins, and extraradicular infections often harbor bacteria and present themselves as chronically and intermittently symptomatic teeth. Apical surgery can be performed to eradicate such factors (Figs. 5.4 through 5.6).

Exploratory Surgery

In certain cases, it may be difficult to properly diagnose a problem. In cases of root fractures, for example, a small soft tissue flap followed by dying the area in question with methylene blue and inspection under the SOM can quickly reveal a root fracture, which can then prevent unnecessary endodontic treatment to be performed on a nonrestorable tooth (Figs. 5.7 and 5.8).

Also, collection of a biopsy specimen may be another indication for performing an exploratory surgery.

CONTRAINDICATIONS FOR ENDODONTIC SURGERY

Medical History

Patients with recent myocardial infarction, with uncontrolled diabetes, patients who are under anticoagulant therapy, patients who received head and neck radiation, or patients with severe neutropenia are not good candidates for surgery. Surgery should be postponed until they are cleared by their treating physician.

Compromised Periodontium

Periodontal pockets and tooth mobility reduce the success of endodontic surgery. High success rates in endodontic microsurgery was achieved in studies where the prospective teeth did not exhibit any pathologic periodontal pocketing or pocketing that either communicated with the apical endodontic component or had completely denuded the buccal or lingual cortical plate of bone resulting in a dehiscence (Rubinstein and Kim 1999).

Skill, Knowledge, and Proper Instruments

General practitioners must be knowledgeable to properly diagnose and refer patients with surgical needs to surgeons who have the specialized training in diagnosing and treating these cases.

Although the skill levels of the surgeons should theoretically be the same, in reality this may not be the case. A study reviewed the outcome of treatment in the oral surgical and endodontics departments of a teaching hospital 4 years following surgery. Complete healing for cases performed by the endodontic unit was nearly twice as high for those performed in the oral surgery unit. The single most important contributing factor was the quality of the procedure, which in turn translated into the surgeon's skill and perhaps level of training and understanding of the problem at hand (Rahbaran 2001).

Despite the surgeon's highest level of clinical competence, proper instrumentation is required for achieving the highest level of technical excellence. It may sound anecdotal, but it is impractical for a world class skier to win any race while skiing on tennis rackets!

Finally, surgeons must keep the welfare of the patient in mind at all times. Case selection for surgery is very important, and indiscriminant use of surgeries to treat endodontic problems is discouraged. Remember, just because you can, does not mean you should (Figs. 5.9 and 5.10).

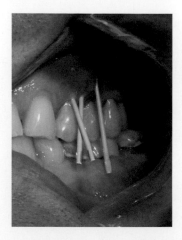

Fig. 5.7. Multiple sinus tracts trace to the location of the endodontic lesion.

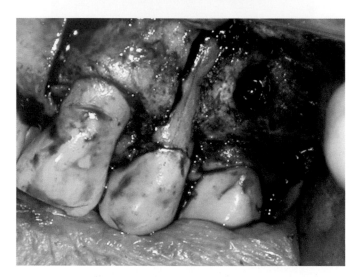

Fig. 5.8. An exploratory surgery and staining reveal a vertical root fracture.

Anatomical Challenges

Proximity to the maxillary sinus, mental nerve, and inferior alveolar canal and the thickness of the buccal bone in the mandibular second molar area due to the external oblique ridge may serve as a contraindication or deterrent for surgery. As long as a properly trained clinician is aware of such hurdles and conceivably knows how to work around them and manage midprocedure and postprocedure potential complications, these factors may be downgraded to potential risks or contraindications. Extra caution or modifications in the procedure may be required in order to avoid damage to such structures.

As an example, the roots of many maxillary molars and premolars are separated from the maxillary sinus by a thin layer of cortical bone and the Schneiderian membrane. Care must be taken not to violate this space. However, in the event that the sinus is inadvertently perforated, with proper care, the

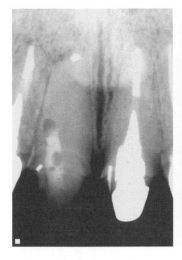

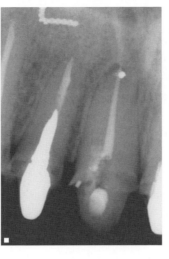

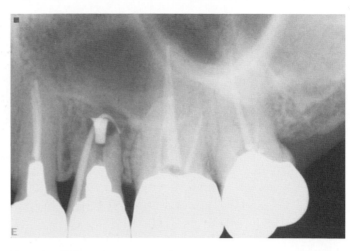

Fig. 5.9. Apicoectomy was performed on a "calcified" central incisor without treating the tooth by nonsurgical root canal therapy first.

Fig. 5.10. Nonsurgical root canal treatment was performed with the aid of the SOM. The tooth was free of symptoms thereafter.

Fig. 5.12. Failing apicoectomy and sinus tract tracing in a maxillary second premolar.

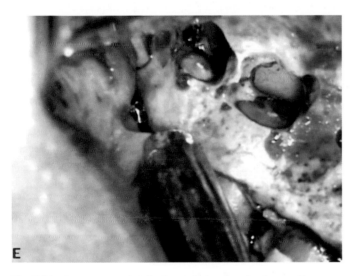

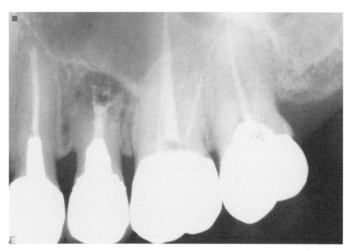

Fig. 5.11. Osteotomy and stained resected root ends of a maxillary molar. Note the maxillary sinus and its lining deep to the root tips.

Fig. 5.13. Conservative apicoectomy and obturation with MTA was performed despite the unfavorable crown-to-root ratio.

membrane usually heals uneventfully, without any negative effect on the outcome of the apical surgery (Fig. 5.11).

Inadequate Root Length

As a critical part of thorough treatment planning, the length of the root before surgery must be estimated. This will allow the clinician to have an understanding whether a favorable crown to root ratio is achievable once the root is resected. If the length of the root after resection is conceived to be inadequate, this may be ground for aborting the surgical procedure and looking for an alternative plan. Although, in select cases where patient is free of periodontal disease, parafunctional habits, and malocclusion, teeth have been known to survive with as low as 1:1 crown-to-root ratio (Figs. 5.12 through 5.14).

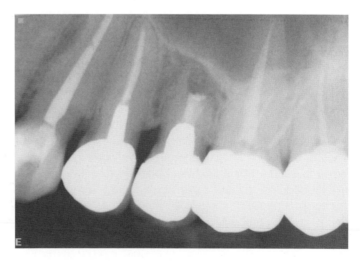

Fig. 5.14. Five-year recall revealed complete healing with no signs of the sinus tract or presence of mobility.

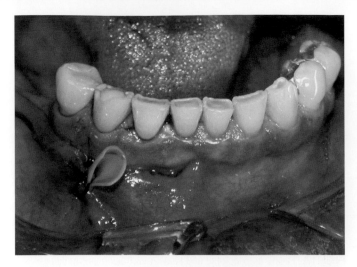

Fig. 5.15. Incision and drainage of an intraoral abscess. Note the latex drain was sutured to prevent its premature removal.

TYPES OF ENDODONTIC SURGERY

Incision and Drainage

Incision and drainage is used for treating necrotic teeth with acute apical abscess. After primary drainage through the tooth is established by performing a pulpectomy, a small incision is made at the base of the fluctuant swelling. Blunt dissection with a curved hemostat facing the bone plate is carried out to dissect tissue plains and establish further drainage. A drain must be placed for up to 48 hours to prevent wound closure. Keeping the incision site open will ensure continuous drainage and patient comfort by allowing the pressure to be relieved (Fig. 5.15).

In addition, by allowing oxygen to gain access to the site of infection, the anaerobic bacteria are killed, the balance of bacteria colony is disrupted, and the rate of healing may be accelerated.

Root Amputation and Hemisection

Root amputation and hemisection involve surgical removal and surgical division of roots of multirooted teeth. Although once performed more frequently, with the increased prevalence of dental implants, the frequency is declining. It is preferred that if a tooth is treatment planned for either of these two procedures, the root canal treatment is performed before the surgical phase. It should be noted that with proper case selection, both procedures are viable options for maintaining the natural teeth. As prudent dentists, we must subdue our urges to perform "herodontics" at all cost in order to maintain a tooth in the oral cavity. Teeth that may serve as strategic abutments, exhibit advanced periodontitis or nonrestorable

remaining segment, and have fused roots or very low furcations are not good candidates for these types of surgery.

Intentional Replantation

As defined by Dr. Grossman, replantation is "the purposeful removal of a tooth and its almost immediate replacement with the object of obturating the canals apically while the tooth is out of its socket" (Kim 2001). Intentional replantation is an artificial setting mimicking complete tooth avulsion, and its management as defined by the guidelines of the American Association of Endodontists. However, the circumstancing factors are near ideal. The level of tooth contamination and physical damage is likely to be far less than in the case of an accidental injury. Moreover, the single most important factor in the demise of an avulsed tooth, the extraoral dry time, is not a factor because it is practically nonexistent. During intentional replantation, the tooth is immediately submerged in tissue culture medium, with the tooth out-of-socket times being under 10 minutes.

The procedure dates back to the late 1500s, when Paré replanted three avulsed teeth (Kupfer 1952). Intentional replantation has been performed for over half a century with success rates being reported between 80% and 95% for follow-ups of 2 to 22 years by Grossman, Kingsbury, and Bender (Kim 2001). Although many of these teeth exhibited some degree of ankylosis and replacement resorption, they were clinically functional and did not exhibit any signs of periradicular pathosis. With the development of new protocols that call for the use of Hanks balanced salt solution (HBSS) (BioWhittaker, Walkersville, MD, USA) as an intermediate storage and operating medium, and the use of enamel matrix derived protein (Emdogain; Straumann, Waldenburg, Switzerland) along with careful extraction techniques to prevent damage to the cementum and the PDL cells, the chances of resorption can be minimized.

Indications and Case Selection

Intentional replantation should not be the treatment of choice if endodontic retreatment or surgery can be performed with a foreseeable positive outcome. Intentional replantation may be considered to be the treatment of choice for treatment of cases where surgical access to the site is impractical or impossible. Teeth with root perforations in mesial, distal, or furcal regions are great candidates. Teeth with expected elaborate apical anatomy and portals of exit or teeth where the apices are lying deep within the jaw bone and surgical access is difficult are also good candidates.

Case selection in intentional replantation plays a big role on the success of the treatment. Teeth with conical fused roots are generally good candidates because of their ease of extraction. On the other hand, teeth with periodontal involvement, thick interseptal bone, or dilacerated roots are contraindicated for intentional replantation.

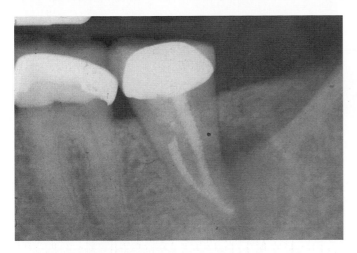

Fig. 5.16. Mandibular second molar exhibiting persistent radiolucency even after nonsurgical retreatment.

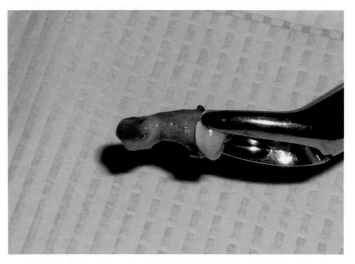

Fig. 5.17. Tooth extraction without placing the forceps on root structure. Note the lesion attached at the root's apical third.

Surgical Technique

After proper case selection and review of the medical history, local anesthesia is administered via block and local infiltration to properly anesthetize the patient. The patient should start to rinse with 10 mL of 0.12% chlorohexidine gluconate twice daily 24 hours before the surgery and continue this regimen for 1 week following the procedure. Although somewhat of a controversy, some advocate the administration of prophylactic antibiotics 24 hours before and for 1 week after the procedure. It is also recommended that unless the patient is allergic to NSAIDs, the maximum daily dose of a drug such as ibuprofen should be prescribed and taken 24 hours before and for 1 week after the procedure. Once the patient is seated and anesthetized, it is crucial to make sure that every step of the procedure is well thought of and ready to be executed. Organization translates into minimized out-of-socket time (less than 10 minutes) and, in turn, maximizes the potential for a successful outcome. After administration of local anesthesia, the tooth can be prepared by working a periotome circumferentially into the gingival sulcus to dissect the fibers. Great care must be taken not to scrape the cementum covering the root surface. Luxation with universal forceps placed only on the anatomical crown is followed. At no time should the beaks of the forceps be making contact with any portion of the tooth apical to the CEJ (cementoenamel junction) (Figs. 5.16 and 5.17).

The use of elevators is contraindicated. It is critical to be extra cautious during this step of the procedure, as a careful and minimally traumatic extraction could be the rate determining step for the outcome. It is not unusual to take as long as 15 minutes to have the tooth fully avulsed. Forcing the extraction could ultimately fracture the tooth or the alveolus and be the demise. Once the tooth is extracted, the crown may firmly be wrapped with sterile gauze and grabbed tightly with a locking hemostat. Curettage of the socket is not recommended.

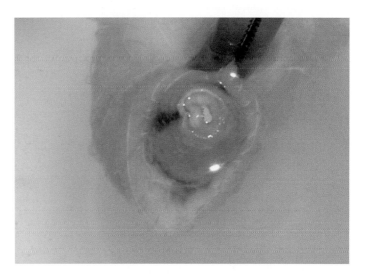

Fig. 5.18. Tooth wrapped in sterile gauze and submerged in HBSS. Root resection was carried out by an Impact air 45 high-speed handpiece.

Making contact with the root surface should be avoided at all times. The tooth is immediately transferred into a basin which is filled with HBSS and submerged. Root resection is carried out by an impact air handpiece under the microscope and approximately 3 mm of the root is resected (Fig. 5.18).

Methylene blue stain is applied to the root end and observed under the microscope with mid-range magnification for cracks, isthmuses, and extra portals of exit. Retropreparation is made by using small pear-shaped carbide burs such as a 330 bur or ultrasonic tips. The canals are then obturated with super ethoxybenzoic acid (Super-EBA; Bosworth, Skokie, IL, USA) or MTA carried in microcarriers and condensed with

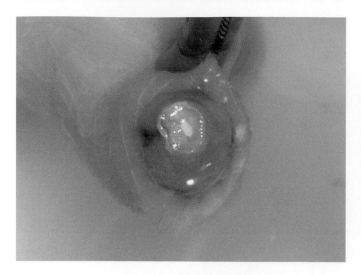

Fig. 5.19. White MTA retrofill.

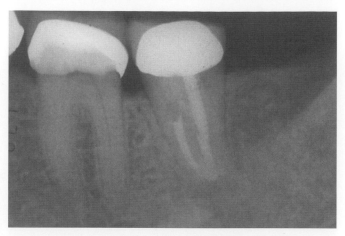

Fig. 5.21. Two-year recall exhibits complete healing.

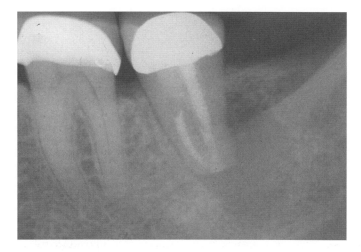

Fig. 5.20. Radiograph immediately post reimplantation

micropluggers. The root end is then polished or burnished and inspected one last time under the microscope before replantation (Fig. 5.19).

The tooth is then reoriented properly and gently placed in its socket. Light apical pressure is applied until the tooth is seated in its correct, most apical position. It is prudent to radiographically confirm the complete seating of the tooth in the socket at this time (Fig. 5.20).

The tooth is then splinted by suturing a monofilament suture over the occlusal surface of the tooth. Fishing line and composite bonding can also be used by providing a physiological splint when the treated tooth is splinted to its neighbor on their buccal surfaces. The limitation of this method is that it requires both of the teeth being splinted to have enamel on their buccal surfaces to facilitate bonding. This method excludes teeth

with metal or porcelain coronal coverage, which may be a good number of teeth treated by intentional replantation. The patient should be instructed to maintain a maximum intercuspal position at least for the remainder of the day and to chew away from the side for about 1 week. Postoperative instructions are given and the patient should be reappointed for follow-up visit in 1 week, at which time the sutures are removed if still intact. Pain management instructions are given as described earlier. Once regarded as a last resort before extraction, today intentional replantation in selected cases is a viable and logical mode of treatment. With the development of new protocols for intentional replantation, the procedure has become more predictable and should always be considered as a part of possible treatment planning (Fig. 5.21).

PERIRADICULAR SURGERY

Periradicular surgeries, otherwise known as apicoectomy, constitute the bulk of endodontic surgeries. By definition, *apicoectomy* involves the reflection of a soft tissue flap, osteotomy of both cortical and cancellous bone, and resection of the root segment, which is suspected to be associated with a persistent inflammatory process. The preparation of a retrocavity and placement of a root-end filling material are not necessary requirements for an apicoectomy, although they are highly recommended. Apicoectomy is perceived to be technically more difficult than other endodontic surgeries due to difficulties in its accessibility, illumination, and small operating field. This is especially true with the case of posterior teeth, that the access more than the anatomy renders them more difficult to treat (Wang 2004). However, since the addition of the SOM to our arsenal of armamentarium, we have been able to overcome many of the challenges associated with apicoectomy.

Indications

Apicoectomy is indicated for treatment of teeth with persistent apical or periradicular pathosis due to anatomical chal-

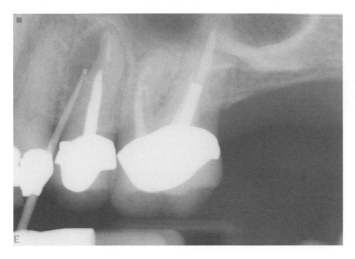

Fig. 5.22. Sinus tract tracing and the location of the mid-root radiolucency is suggestive of a post perforation.

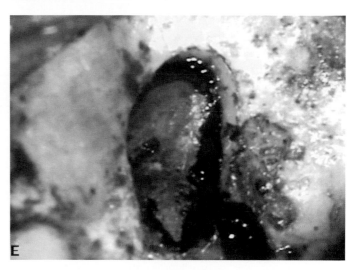

Fig. 5.24. Staining reveals a perforation on the mesial aspect of the root. The defect was filled with Super-EBA cement.

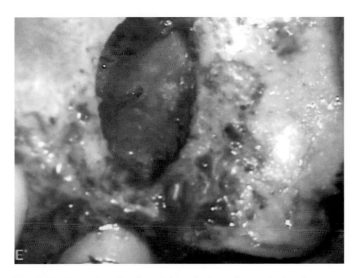

Fig. 5.23. Upon the reflection of the soft tissue flap, an isolated endodontic fenestration is visible.

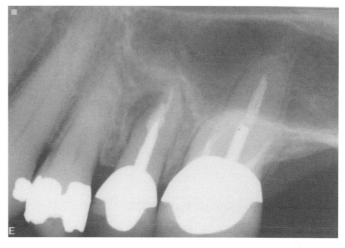

Fig. 5.25. A 3-month recall revealed partial healing and no signs of the sinus tract.

lenges, iatrogenic factors, irretrievable dental material inside and outside of the canal, fractures, and repair of resorptions or perforations (Figs. 5.22 to 5.25).

PHASES OF APICOECTOMY AND SURGICAL TECHNIQUE

Review of Medical History

Once the patient has been selected as a candidate for apical surgery, a complete review of the systemic health of the patient must be performed. High-risk patients as defined by the American Heart Association are to be pretreated prophylactically with oral antibiotics. After consultation with their physician, patients who are on anticoagulant therapy should be

taken off of the medication in time before the surgery. Last, patients who have been on oral or intravenous bisphosphonates should be informed about the potential risks and complications that may arise after the surgery as sequelae of the drug therapy.

Intraoral Examination

A thorough intraoral examination is crucial in postulating and designing the appropriate approach for treatment via surgery. Intraorally, the surgical site should be investigated for any type of periodontal defect by careful probing. Evaluation of periodontal recession, width of attached gingiva, and the patient's gingival biotype may ultimately determine the type of incision used during the surgery. Any sinus tracts, swellings, or areas sensitive to palpation should be noted. Evaluation of muscle attachments and patient's opening are critical in determining accessibility to the prospective surgical site.

Radiographic Examination

Exposure of two periapical radiographs is the minimum requirement before commencement of surgery. The first radiograph should be exposed using a paralleling technique and the second should be deviated in its horizontal component by 20 degrees to the mesial or distal. The radiograph should be studied for root length, number of roots, root curvature, size of the potential lesion, and proximity of the osteotomy to neurovascular bundles, maxillary sinus, and neighboring teeth. It is strongly recommended that, when possible, a panoramic radiograph is obtained, especially when treating mandibular posterior teeth.

Presurgical Preparation

Preoperatively, unless contraindicated, the patient should take 600 to 800 mg of ibuprofen just before surgery. The patient should continue to take this regimen of anti-inflammatory every 8 hours for up to 3 days after the surgery.

In addition, the patient should commence rinsing with 10 mL of 0.12% chlorohexidine gluconate twice daily, 24 hours before surgery. This oral rinse should be used before surgery to reduce the quantity of the microorganisms in the mouth and decrease the chance of a postsurgical flap infection.

Local Anesthesia (Pain Control and Hemostasis)

Choosing and administering the appropriate local anesthetic has a trifold effect. First, it provides pain control during the surgery. Second, it provides hemostasis. Third, by administering a long-lasting anesthetic, postoperatively, the cycle of pain is broken. This is in part due to prevention in amplification of responses from the peripheral nerves, which could ultimately lead to central sensitization.

Typically, local anesthesia is administered via nerve blocks and local infiltrations. Nerve blocks are aimed at achieving profound pain control but must be supplemented by local infiltrations and papillary injections on both the buccal and lingual aspects of the teeth for additional pain control and hemostasis.

Unless contraindicated, 2% lidocaine with 1:50,000 epinephrine is the anesthetic of choice because of its high concentration of epinephrine, which is suitable for hemostasis. Although this high concentration of epinephrine may cause a transient tachycardia in the patient, the effects are generally short lived. It should be noted that some clinicians prefer 3%

Marcaine with epinephrine for nerve block because of its long duration of action.

In addition to the administration of one cartridge of anesthetic for the appropriate nerve block when working on maxillary or mandibular teeth, local infiltration into oral tissue for hemostasis is required. Generally, up to two cartridges of anesthetic should be infiltrated locally around two or three teeth on either side of the surgical site. Because most of the receptors in the masticatory mucosa are of α–adrenergic type, once bound to epinephrine, they produce a desired vasoconstrictive effect. In contrast, because the majority of the receptors in skeletal muscles are of the β_2–adrenergic variety and their binding to epinephrine causes vasodialation, care must be taken to prevent injecting deep into these tissues.

Soft Tissue Flap Design

Proper flap design not only should provide easy access to the location of the pathosis but also should consider and provide postsurgical aesthetics of the periodontium and the gingiva, especially preserving marginal gingiva and papillary heights. With the evolution of periodontal surgery and introduction of new techniques, some older techniques have been phased out.

Periodontal condition of the failing tooth and its neighboring teeth play an important role in the design of the soft tissue flap; so does the prosthetic state of the surgical site. When working on teeth with crowns or areas near the pontic of a fixed partial denture, modifications to the incision line may be needed to facilitate suturing and ensure soft tissue aesthetics in the long term. Also of importance are anatomical factors, such as the mental foramen, which may ultimately play a role in the selection of the location for the placement of the vertical release incision.

In endodontic surgery, incisions are made to facilitate elevation and reflection of a full-thickness flap. Generally, a horizontal component and two vertical release incisions are used to provide easy access without pulling and tearing the corners of the flap. Once the tissue is reflected, great care must be taken to prevent the placement of the retractors on soft tissue. Many manufacturers have developed contour specific retractors that provide good ergonomic retraction of the flap in different locations of the mouth. In some cases, slipping of the retractor can be prevented by placing a notch or a groove superficially on the cortical bone and subsequently placing the retractor in this groove.

The following is a list of flaps that are associated with endodontic surgery:

Semilunar Incision

Although once frequently used by endodontists and oral surgeons for performing apicoectomies, semilunar incisions are an inferior and obsolete technique. Typically, they provide poor access to the site and do not allow for addressing or treating periodontal–endodontic involvements. They often result in unsightly scars as the incision line is made in unattached, mobile oral mucosa, and over the osteotomy where healing by primary intention is impractical, if not impossible.

Today, semilunar incisions are performed only during emergency incision and drainage.

Full-Thickness Intrasulcular Incision

In this technique, the horizontal incision commences at the base of the gingival sulcus and is carried through to the crest of the bone by dissecting the periodontal ligament fibers. Generally, the horizontal component should be extended by the width of two teeth on either side of the tooth being treated. Interproximally, the incision should be made with a sharp 15C or a CK-2 microblade (Sybron Endo, Orange, CA, USA) lingually while following the contour of the teeth. The complete dissection of the interdental papilla before elevation is desired to prevent recession and formation of "black triangles" postoperatively.

Two variations of the full thickness intrasulcular flap exist:

- The triangular flap, which uses one vertical releasing incision in the more medial aspect of the flap, typically requires a longer horizontal incision. The releasing incision should begin perpendicular to the line of the free gingival margin for a short distance of approximately 2 to 3 mm. It is then rounded off at the corner and transitioned into the vertical component of the releasing incision. It is not unusual to extend the release incision up to the mucobuccal fold and up to 2 times the length of release incisions in periodontal surgery in order to access the root apex easily. Triangular flaps are commonly used in surgeries of the posterior region

(Figs. 5.26 to 5.28), or in the anterior region when treating teeth with cervical resorptions or perforations.

- The rectangular flap is similar to the triangular flap, except it uses two vertical releasing incisions and as a result, the horizontal incision may be shorter. This flap provides better access to the apex of anterior teeth than the triangular flap.

Full-Thickness Submarginal Incision

Also known as the mucogingival flap, it is indicated primarily in anterior surgeries to treat teeth with crowns and where aesthetics of the crown margin is of a great deal of importance. The beveled scalloped horizontal component of the incision is placed in attached gingiva and is terminated by rounding off and transitioning into the placement of two parallel vertical releasing incisions at either end. The scalloping aids in exact repositioning of the flap postsurgically to ensure

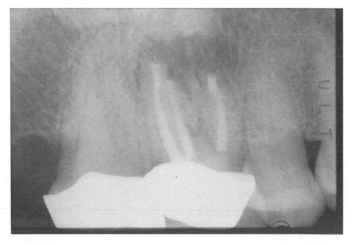

Fig. 5.27. Triangular full-thickness flap provides access to the surgical site.

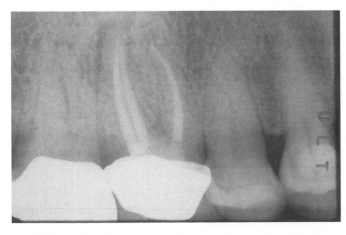

Fig. 5.26. Maxillary first molar exhibiting persistent symptoms despite the radiographically acceptable appearance of the nonsurgical root canal therapy.

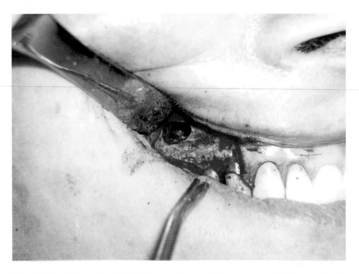

Fig. 5.28. Apicoectomy and retrofill with MTA was performed on all three roots via a buccal approach.

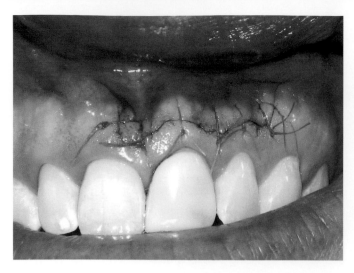

Fig. 5.29. Submarginal incision and suturing with 6-0 Vicryl sutures in the aesthetic zone.

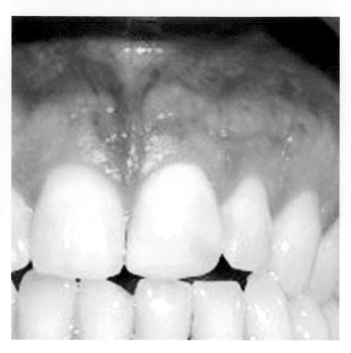

Fig. 5.30. Suture removal 4 days later reveals great healing with minimal scar formation.

healing by primary intention. It is critical to have a 2-mm band of healthy attached gingiva coronal and apical to the horizontal incision line (Figs. 5.29 and 5.30).

Lack of such attachment especially coronal to the incision may critically undermine the blood supply and result in disastrous postsurgical recession. Needless to say, acquiring accurate preoperative periodontal probing depths is critical.

This flap differs from the Luebke-Ochsenbein flap in that it is not wider at the base because the two vertical releasing incisions are made parallel to each other.

Papillary-Based Incision

This technique has been developed in recent years with the purpose of maintaining the height of the interdental papilla. The incision is similar to the full-thickness intrasulcular incision. However, in the region of the interdental papilla, instead of the incision including and dissecting the papilla, it is placed at the base of the papilla. This incision is a curved incision that connects the sulcus of one tooth at its mesial line angle to the sulcus of the more anterior tooth at its distal line angle. This incision is carried out by a microblade first to a depth of 1.5 mm. A second incision is directed toward the osseous crest and retraces the initial superficial incision.

Upon completion of the surgery, proper suturing is important to guarantee optimal results. Generally, the use of 7-0 or smaller monofilament nonresorbable sutures has been recommended for closure of the papillary based incision. A minimum of two single interrupted sutures are placed to ensure primary closure at the papillary base. Sutures are to be removed within 3 to 5 days (Velvart and Peters 2005).

Osteotomy and Curettage

Once the flap is reflected and stabilized without causing trauma to the soft tissue, the hard tissue management phase of the surgery may begin. The root tip location must be approximated from a preoperative radiograph, presence of pathology, cortical bone fenestration, or a root prominence underlying the cortical bone. In some cases sounding the bone quality over the root apex with a sharp endodontic DG16 explorer (Hu-Friedy, Chicago, IL, USA) may give information about the location and the extent of the underlying lesion (Figs. 5.31 and 5.32).

Once the location for the osteotomy is determined, using an Impact Air 45 (Palisades Dental, Englewood, NJ, USA) high-speed handpiece and Lindemann H 161 (Brasseler USA, Savannah, GA, USA) bone-cutting carbide bur, the osteotomy is made under low magnification with copious irrigation with sterile saline to cool the surgical site. This is done by brushing away at the bone until the root apex is visualized (Fig. 5.33).

With the advent of modern microsurgical instruments, the ideal osteotomy can now be only 5 mm in diameter.

Any soft tissue lesion attached to the root tip must be curettaged before root resection. This is achieved by the back action use of long shank spoon excavators or bone curettes to detach the lesion from its bony housing in total. This tis-

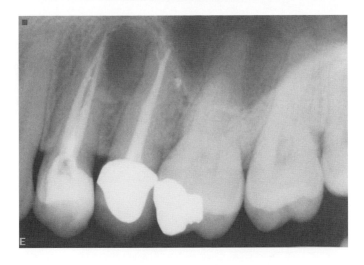

Fig. 5.31. Failing root canal treatment on maxillary first and second premolars.

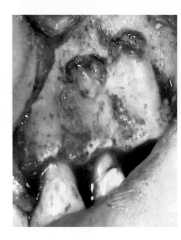

Fig. 5.33. Osteotomy is initiated by slow removal of the buccal cortical bone until the root tips are visible.

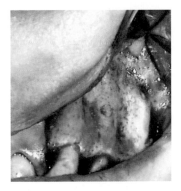

Fig. 5.32. Flap elevation reveals fenestrations over the root prominences identifying the location of the defects.

sue must be submitted for biopsy. Any remnants still attached to the root can be removed via a 34/35 Jaquette scaler or a 13/14 periodontal curette (Hu-Friedy). Excessive curettage of the bony crypt may cause excessive bleeding, which may in turn complicate and compromise the stages of root-end resection, retropreparation, and retrofilling. Therefore, it may be more strategic to leave small amounts of granulation tissue behind and clean it after the root-end filling is placed.

The Impact Air 45 high-speed handpiece is designed in such way that only a water coolant is sprayed out from the front onto the bur. The air jet is contained within a closed circuit and ejected from the rear of the handpiece. This innovation allows for a much cleaner operation due to the lack of splatter previously caused by the air stream forced out of the head of conventional handpieces. Most important, it creates a safer operation by eliminating the air that may be forced into the open vessels of the surgical site and potentially cause an air emphysema.

Root Resection

The logic behind root resection and its extent is derived from the models developed by Hess. A 3-mm reduction in the root end will decrease the incidence of lateral canals by 93% and apical ramifications by 98%. Therefore statistically, a 3-mm apicoectomy will markedly favor the elimination of persistent bacteria and undebrided tissue in the apical root canal portion (Kim 2001). This will also enable the surgeon to remove and eliminate iatrogenic factors more prevalent to the last 2 to 3 mm of the root canal system. Once the root is resected, access to the canal is possible for evaluation and formation of an impervious retroseal.

Up until the early 1990s, the practice was to resect the root end with a 45-degree buccolingual bevel. This was practiced because it was impossible to form a cavity preparation into the canal even with the smallest handpiece. Presently, with the development of microsurgical instruments, and, more specifically, ultrasonic tips, micromirrors, and pluggers, the recommended root-end resection bevel angle is between 0 and 10 degrees. This modification in technique has its many advantages. It conserves root and buccal cortical bone and reduces the chance of incomplete resection and perhaps missing lingual anatomy. By reducing the cavity preparation, cavosurface margin, and number of exposed dentinal tubules, the risk of microleakage is reduced (Kim 2002).

This phase of the procedure should be carried out under mid-range magnification using the Impact Air 45 handpiece and

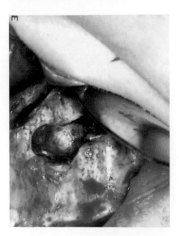

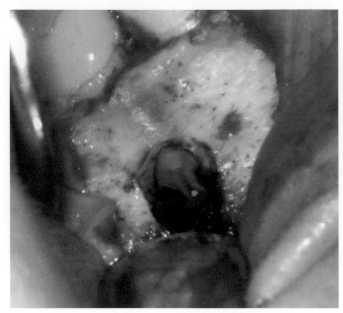

Fig. 5.34. Endodontic lesion is enucleated in whole and the root tips are resected with almost a zero bevel angle.

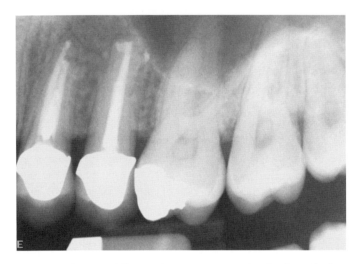

Fig. 5.36. The resected and stained mesial root of a mandibular molar reveals an unfilled MB canal and the isthmus connecting the MB and ML canals.

Fig. 5.35. One-year follow-up demonstrates complete healing of both teeth.

Lindemann H 161 bur with sterile saline irrigation (Figs. 5.34 and 5.35).

Staining and Inspection

Once the root end is perceived as being completely resected, it is time to switch the magnification to the high range for root-end inspection. The root end should be stained with sterile methylene blue dye (American Regent Inc., Shirley, NY, USA) and rinsed away with sterile saline or water. The dye will stain the PDL circumferentially, revealing a circle or an ovoid blue perimeter. This is a sign that the root resection was completely carried out through the lingual aspect. The blue dye will also penetrate into any canal, isthmus, portal of exit, or fracture and reveal areas that need to be prepared with the ultrasonic tips (Fig. 5.36).

Prior to the use of ultrasonic tips, a CX-1 microexplorer (Sybron EndoA) may be used to probe into these areas. Sometimes it is helpful to scribe the preparation outline with the CX-1 onto the root-end surface before the use of ultrasonic tips.

Retropreparation

After the areas to be retroprepared have been identified, ultrasonic tips with the appropriate angulations can be used to create the cavity preparation along the long axis of the root. This step should also be carried out under high magnification and constant irrigation. Incorporating the isthmus between two canals or a fin to the side of a canal into the preparation is just as critical as preparing the canals themselves (Figs. 5.37 to 5.39).

Any tissue left in the isthmus could be a source for a potential failure. The preparation is carried out to a depth of 3 to 4 mm. The preparation should be inspected under the microscope in order to ensure that no gutta percha remains on the prepared portion of the canal walls. A microplugger/condenser can be used to compact any residual gutta percha coronally and away from the root tip.

Some surgeons prefer to treat the root end with a 2% chlorohexidine gluconate (Ultradent, South Jordan, UT, USA). This antibacterial agent has proved to be effective against *E. faecalis,* the persistent bacteria species in many endodontic failures.

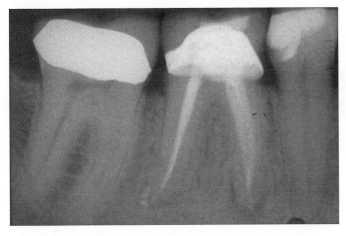

Fig. 5.37. Mandibular first molar exhibiting persistent pathology of the mesial root.

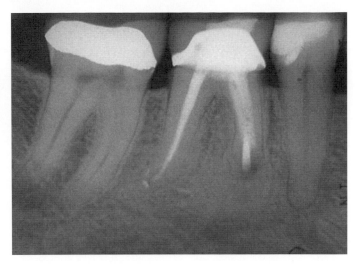

Fig. 5.39. Near-complete healing is noted at 6-month recall appointment.

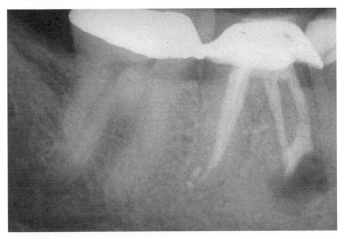

Fig. 5.38. Apicoectomy, retropreparation, and retrofill of the MB and ML canals and the isthmus connecting them.

Moisture Control

The bone crypt must be dry before the placement of the retrofill material. If bleeding is present, it may be controlled by the application of topical hemostatic agents. Racellet #3 (Pascal Co., Bellevue, WA, USA) epinephrine pellets are usually effective in controlling the bleeding in most osteotomy sites. They contain racemic epinephrine, which aid in hemostasis. These pellets are packed into the osteotomy site with moderate pressure maintained on them for a few minutes. Once hemostasis is achieved, all but the last of the pellets are removed. The last pellet is deliberately left in the crypt to maintain the hemostasis. Aspiration into the crypt once hemostasis has been achieved should be prevented, because it may draw blood out of the capillaries and initiate bleeding again. It is important to keep track of the number of pellets placed, so at the end of the procedure, pellets are not forgotten and left behind.

For more persistent bleeding in larger osteotomies, ferric sulfate solution such as Cut-Trol (Ichthys Inc., Mobile, AL, USA) may be used. Ferric sulfate has been shown to delay postoperative healing (Lemon 1993). Therefore, it should only be used sparingly and curettaged and rinsed thoroughly at the end of the surgery before suturing.

Calcium sulfate such as Surgiplast (ClassImplant, Rome, Italy) can also be used as a mechanical barrier to promote hemostasis in large osteotomies. Calcium sulfate is an osteoinductive resorbable agent that may act as a barrier against the more rapid mobilization of soft tissue cells towards the osteotomy site and, therefore, promote bone formation.

Retrofill

Once the moisture is controlled, it is time for sealing the root end. The root end must be irrigated and air dried with a Stropko irrigator/drier with a microtip (Sybron Endo).

Although amalgam was once the root-end filling of choice, today it is no longer the standard of care to place amalgam as a retrograde filling. Today's materials provide a better seal, do not tattoo the gingiva, do not corrode, and are more biocompatible than amalgam. Although an array of materials are presently available, MTA and Super-EBA are the most promising and most widely used.

MTA exhibits many of the desired characteristics of a retrofill material. MTA is radiopaque and gentle to the periapical tissue, induces cementogenesis, has great sealing ability, and is tolerant to moisture. In fact, MTA requires moisture to harden and set. Unfortunately, it is difficult to handle. MTA is mixed with sterile water to form a wet sand–like granular mixture. The easiest way to place it into the root-end preparation is with the MAP System (Roydent, Johnson City, TN, USA) or the MTA pellet forming block (G. Hartzell & Son, Concord, CA, USA). Once placed, MTA takes a long time to set and should not be rinsed out. The crypt may be cleaned with a moist cotton pellet.

Super-EBA, on the other hand, is difficult to mix but easier to handle. It is mixed into a hard, dull, dough-like mixture by incorporating powder into liquid with a thick spatula over a glass slab. Once ready, time is limited to place it because it sets quickly, especially in the presence of heat and humidity. Super-EBA is rolled into a small cone and picked up in small segments with an instrument such as a Hollenbeck or the back side of a spoon excavator. It is then placed into the root end, compacted gently with a microplugger, and finally burnished with a microball burnisher. After the material is fully set, it may be polished with a composite finishing bur using a high speed handpiece with irrigation.

Once the retrofill material is placed, it is a good practice to radiographically verify the density and the depth of the fill before suturing the flap. If any modifications need to be made, this is a good time for it.

After the quality of the filling is confirmed to be satisfactory, the crypt must be curettaged to remove any residual material or coagulum and to induce bleeding. The surgical site should be rinsed with sterile saline to wash off any particles or loose debris and also to rehydrate the flap and the cortical bone, which may have been drying under the intense illumination from the SOM.

Suturing and Suture Removal

The flap needs to be reapproximated passively before suturing. Best results are obtained when the flap margins approximate without the use of force or under tension. For this purpose, a wet 2 × 2 guaze is compressed gently over the flap and cortical bone until tissue margins assume their preferred position.

As for suture material, monofilament nonresorbable Prolene (Ethicon Inc., Somerville, NJ, USA) sutures in sizes of 6-0 or smaller provide the optimal results. The advantage of these types of sutures is that their size causes the least amount of trauma and that they are nonresorbable, which minimizes the inflammation typically associated with suture materials. When suturing the apical margins of the vertical release incision near the mucobuccal fold, however, it is advantageous to use a resorbable suture such as a coated Vicryl or Monocryl (Ethicon Inc.). Sutures in this region sometimes have a tendency to become imbedded into the wound closure and may be difficult to remove.

In terms of suturing technique, single interrupted and vertical mattress sutures are the most commonly used. Vertical mattress sutures are preferred when suturing mobilized interdental papillae in the anterior esthetic zone. Sling sutures in the posterior region can be used in place of two single interrupted sutures. When suturing the vertical releasing incision, a continuous interlocking suture can be used to expedite suturing by eliminating the need for multiple knots.

Whatever the suturing technique, care must be taken that the suture and the knots are free of any tension. Tissue margins may be torn when sutures are tight and act as a guillotine. In addition, the underlying tissue may become deprived of blood perfusion and ultimately necrose in presence of overtighten knots.

Postsurgically, sutures should be removed within 3 to 5 days, although some studies advocate suture removal by 48 hours.

Postoperative Instructions

Postoperative instructions should be directed toward ensuring patient's comfort, control of bleeding and swelling, and prevention of infections.

Patient reassurance is an important part of postoperative instructions. It is better for the patient to know about potential pain, swelling, or bruising ahead of time rather than being caught by surprise.

Pain following endodontic surgery is usually mild. For this reason non-narcotic analgesics are more than adequate in controlling patient's pain. Just before the start of the procedure, 1000 mg of acetaminophen or 800 mg of ibuprofen should be taken by the patient as a preemptive strike against pain when the local anesthetic slowly wears off. Postsurgically, ibuprofen 800 mg three times daily should be prescribed and taken by the patient for 3 to 5 days. This regimen should be followed regardless of the level of patient's comfort as an anti-inflammatory medication. For those patients who are allergic to ibuprofen, 1000 mg acetaminophen can be taken four times daily. Some more recent studies suggest combination therapy with ibuprofen and acetaminophen will achieve more effective levels of analgesia (Menhinick 2004).

Applying an ice pack to the face over the region of surgery with moderate pressure for 20 minutes on and 20 minutes off is very important in controlling inflammation, swelling, and ecchymosis. This regimen is most effective if followed up to 8 hours postsurgically. Moist heat application is recommended for 24 to 48 hours after surgery.

Rinsing with 10 mL of 0.12% chlorohexidine gluconate solution twice daily should begin 24 hours before surgery and continue for up to 2 days after suture removal. Gentle brushing with a soft bristle tooth brush should be limited to the areas away from the surgical site and to the occlusal surfaces of teeth proximal to the incision line.

Patients should be informed that in the event of a suture becoming untied, they should not pull on the loose end as they may detach the flap from the underlying bone.

Consumption of a normal diet is recommended, although a soft diet is preferred for the first 48 hours. In addition, hot liquids should be avoided because they may promote bleeding and cause pain if they become in contact with exposed tissue or bone. Smoking and consumption of alcohol should be avoided until sutures are removed and proper healing is confirmed.

Patients should avoid physical activities that can increase their heart rate and increase bleeding. In addition, patients should be discouraged to manipulate the areas of the face or mouth, which may pull on the sutures and ultimately extricate them.

Complications

Serious complications after endodontic surgery are infrequent. Most cases of pain, swelling, and bleeding are easily managed. In some rare cases, patients may have serious infection or parasthesia. Immediate attention is required for such incidences.

Although parasthesia is often transient and is not due to the complete severing of a nerve bundle, it may cause some concern in the patient. Patients should be reassured that the sensation will often return and it could simply be the result of inflammation and nerve compression. Only in rare occasions is parasthesia irreversible. The patient must be reevaluated at the office, and the affected area must be mapped intraorally by the use of a sharp dental instrument. A diagram of this area must be drawn in the patient's dental record and compared to subsequent examinations to check for signs of improvement. If no improvement is noted, the patient should be referred to a specialist for further care and monitoring.

Infections after endodontic surgery are uncommon. Routine prescription of oral antibiotics is not supported by studies and therefore not recommended. The antibiotic of choice for treating endodontic infections is 500 mg penicillin VK every 6 hours for 1 week. If this initial therapy does not provide the desired pharmaceutical result, it can be supplemented with 500 mg metronidazole every 6 hours for 1 week. Also, the patient can be taken off of the Penicillin VK and placed on 300 mg clindamycin every 8 hours for 1 week. In those rare cases where the patient is severely swollen, febrile, and may have difficulty breathing or swallowing, immediate referral to the hospital and administration of intravenous antibiotics is indicated.

Last, during maxillary posterior surgeries where the maxillary sinus and the Schneiderian membrane have been involved, the patient must be placed on a prophylactic dose of 875 mg of Augmentin twice daily for 1 week to prevent invasion and infection of the sinus by normal oral flora. The patient should also be advised not to blow the nose and to take over-the-counter nasal decongestants. A 1-week follow-up visit is recommended to ensure no complications have arisen. Maxillary sinus involvements, if treated in a timely manner, will often heal uneventfully.

RECALL

Patient's healing must be monitored periodically. Because the average healing time for surgical cases has been reported to be 7 months, it makes sense to recall the patient within 1 year post-treatment. Earlier follow-up appointments may not indicate any healing, although healing may be in progress.

For cases in which a timely secondary intervention would be imperative in case of a failure, a 3- to 4-month recall schedule is justified and perhaps more beneficial.

REFERENCES

ADA 1999 Survey of Dental Services Rendered. ADA Report: September 2002.

Kim, S. Endodontic microsurgery. In S. Cohen and R.C. Burns, editors. *Pathways of the Pulp*, 8th ed. Mosby, St Louis, 2002, pp. 683–725.

Kim, S., G. Pecora, and R. Rubinstein. *Color Atlas of Microsurgery in Endodontics*. WB Saunders, Philadelphia, 2001a, p. 125.

Kim, S., G. Pecora, and R. Rubinstein. *Color Atlas of Microsurgery in Endodontics*. Philadelphia, WB Saunders, 2001b, pp. 85–94.

Kupfer, I.J., R. Sidney, and B.S. Kupfer. 1952. Tooth replantation following avulsion. *N.Y. State Dent. J.* 19:80.

Lemon, R.R., P.J. Steele, and B.G. Jeansonne. 1993. Ferric sulfate hemostasis: effect on osseous wound healing. Left in-situ for maximum exposure. *J. Endod.* 19:170–173.

Menhinick, K., J.L. Gutmann, J.D. Regan, S.E. Taylor, and P.H. Bushang. 2004. The efficacy of pain control following nonsurgical root canal treatment using ibuprofen or a combination of ibuprofen and acetaminophen in a randomized, double-blind, placebo-controlled study. *Int. J. Endod.* 37:531–541.

Rahbaran, S., M.S. Gilthorpe, S.D. Harrison, and K. Gulabivala. 2001. Comparison of clinical outcome of periapical surgery in endodontic and oral surgery units of a teaching dental hospital: a retrospective study. *Oral Surg. Oral Med. Oral Pathol. Oral Radiol. Endod.* 91:700–709.

Reuben, H., and H. Apotheker. 1984. Apical surgery with the dental microscope. *Oral Surg. Oral Med. Oral Pathol.* 57:433–435.

Rubinstein, F.A., and S. Kim. 1999. Short-term observation of the results of endodontic surgery with the use of a surgical operation microscope and Super-EBA as root-end filling material. *J. Endod.* 25:43–48.

Rubinstein, F.A., and S. Kim. 2002. Long-term follow-up of cases considered healed one year after apical microsurgery. *J. Endod.* 28:378–383.

Ruskin, J.D., D. Morton, B. Karayazgan, and J. Amir. 2005. Failed root canals: the case for extraction and immediate implant placement. *J. Oral Maxillofac. Surg.* 63:829–831.

Velvart, P., and C.I. Peters. 2005. Soft tissue management in endodontic surgery. *J. Endod.* 31:4–16.

Wang, N., K. Knight, T. Dao, and S. Friedman. 2004. Treatment outcome in endodontics—the Toronto study. Phase I and II: apical surgery. *J. Endod.* 30:751–761.

Zuolo, M.L., M.O.F. Ferreira, and J.L. Gutmann. 2000. Prognosis in periradicular surgery: a clinical prospective study. *Int. Endod. J.* 33:91–98.

Chapter 6 The Contribution of Periodontics to Prosthodontics: Treatment Planning of Patients Requiring Combined Periodontal and Prosthodontic Care

Haneen N. Bokhadoor, DDS, MSD,

Nawaf J. Al-Dousari, DDS, MSD, and Steven Morgano, DMD

INTRODUCTION

Treatment planning for patients with complex dental needs involves multidisciplinary collaboration with the prosthodontist, periodontist/oral surgeon, orthodontist, endodontist, and patient. It is a carefully sequenced process and is designed to eliminate or control etiologic factors, repair existing damage, and create a functional, maintainable oral environment. Successful treatment depends on a thorough evaluation of all available information, a definitive diagnosis, and a thorough integration of all necessary procedures prescribed for the patient. The treatment process is composed of a series of phases: a diagnostic phase, a treatment-planning phase, a treatment phase, and a maintenance phase.

DIAGNOSTIC PHASE (DATA COLLECTION)

Diagnosis involves the collection of data obtained from a comprehensive patient history (medical and dental), a patient interview (chief complaint), a clinical examination (inspection, palpation and percussion), a critical evaluation of mounted diagnostic casts, and a radiologic interpretation.

Patient History

Patient's Social and Environmental History

The patient's social and environmental history are important adjuncts to diagnosis and treatment planning and can often determine the entire course of treatment. Examples include a patient's age, gender, occupation, alcohol intake, tobacco use, and illicit drug use.

Medical History

The importance of an accurate comprehensive medical history cannot be overstated. The medical history reveals systemic conditions that could be contributing factors related to the existing dental disease or that could affect the prognosis of dental treatment. A thorough medical history and interview should reveal any previous systemic diseases, injuries, surgical procedures, allergies, adverse drug reactions, and medications. An example of a systemic disease affecting oral health is diabetes mellitus. Patients with diabetes mellitus are more likely to develop periodontal disease compared with patients without diabetes, and periodontal disease is often considered the sixth complication of diabetes mellitus. Patients with uncontrolled diabetes are especially at risk (Mealey and Oates 2006).

The medical history can also alert the dentist to other disorders, such as a prosthetic cardiac valve that require antibiotic prophylaxis (Davies 1993). The presence of a pacemaker contraindicates the use of electrosurgery (Flocken 1980). Previous radiation therapy for neoplastic diseases of the head and neck region can have a profound effect on the oral cavity (AAP position paper, 1997). Medications causing xerostomia can lead to cervical dental caries and periodontal disease, and can contribute to early failure of fixed restorations (Thomson et al. 2006). Osteonecrosis of the jaw has been observed in cancer patients who have undergone invasive dental procedures, such as dental implant surgery or tooth extractions, while receiving treatment with intravenous bisphosphonates. Invasive dental procedures should be avoided for these patients whenever possible (Soileau 2006, Wooltorton 2005).

Dental History

The dental history serves as a companion to the medical history. It establishes information on the patient's involvement in previous dental treatment, when and why missing teeth were removed, previous problems with dental treatment, parafunctional habits, and oral hygiene habits.

Chief Complaint

The chief complaint can establish the need for additional diagnostic tests to assist in determining the cause of the dental problems. It is important that any recommended treatment addresses this chief complaint and that the patient's expectations with regard to the outcome of treatment are realistic.

Clinical Examination

Extraoral Examination

A thorough examination should include an evaluation of the size, shape, and symmetry of the head and neck including the patient's profile (retrognathic, mesiognathic, prognathic). Normal and abnormal clinical findings should be noted in detail as a permanent component of the patient's record.

Intraoral Examination

The intraoral examination includes screening for malignancies, an evaluation of the patient's overall caries activity, a general overview of the periodontal status, and the quality and quantity of saliva. The dentist should then thoroughly examine the existing restorations and their status, the presence of dental caries, and missing teeth. A complete periodontal assessment is an important component of a comprehensive oral examination. It includes an evaluation of the oral hygiene, a description of the color, form, and texture of the gingiva, a recording of probing depths, an assessment of bleeding on probing, a determination of tooth mobility, a mucogingival evaluation, and an evaluation of furcations.

Occlusal Examination and Analysis

One of the most critical factors with regard to treatment planning is an evaluation of the patient's occlusion. Alterations and deviations in the occlusal plane can result in a dysfunctional maximal intercuspal position (MIP), attrition, bruxism, widened periodontal ligament spaces (trauma from occlusion), and impaired mastication. Mounted diagnostic casts represent an important diagnostic aid for the thorough evaluation of a patient's occlusion (Morgano et al. 1989).

Radiographic Examination

Basic knowledge of normal radiographic appearances is essential. The minimal examination requirements for a comprehensive treatment plan include a panoramic radiograph and a complete-mouth radiographic series. The presence of dental caries, loss of tooth-supporting bone, furcation invasions, and any other abnormalities should be carefully noted and recorded in the patient's record.

Diagnostic Casts and Diagnostic Waxing

Diagnostic casts are made from impressions of the dental arches. Irreversible hydrocolloid (alginate) material is usually used in stock metal trays. The trays should allow a uniform thickness of 3 to 5 mm of impression material. These trays should be large enough to cover the retromolar pads in the mandible and the hamular (pterygomaxillary) notches in the maxillary arch. The impressions should be poured immediately with cast (Type III) stone. Once the casts are retrieved, small nodules are removed. The casts are mounted in a semiadjustable articulator with a face-bow transfer. Duplicate diagnostic casts are also made and mounted. A diagnostic waxing of the proposed treatment plan is then made. Diagnostic casts and the diagnostic waxing represent the guide or "blueprint" for the restorative plan that assists the dentist and laboratory technician in coordinating the reconstruction of aesthetics, phonetics, and function (Morgano et al. 1989).

Prognosis

The prognosis is a forecast of the probable course and outcome of a disorder. The overall prognosis is concerned with the entire dentition. Criteria used to assign a prognosis to individual teeth are subjective and are usually based on clinical and radiographic findings. A favorable, questionable (guarded), unfavorable (poor) or hopeless prognosis is assigned to each tooth depending on available bone support, probing depths, furcation exposure, mobility, crown-to-root ratio, root proximity, occlusal relationships, extent of tooth damage, abutment status, endodontic status, remaining tooth structure (restorability), caries susceptibility, quality and quantity of saliva, and parafunctional habits.

Making the decision to retain or extract a compromised tooth requires a thorough evaluation of all factors, including the expense and discomfort involved in maintaining the tooth, the overall strategic value of the tooth, available literature from clinical studies on the probability of success of the treatment required to retain the tooth, the prognosis of an artificial replacement for the tooth, and the patient's desires, expectations and needs. Extraction of one or more teeth may be prescribed based on the presence of one or more of the following factors: greater than 75% bone loss, Miller Class III mobility (greater than 1-mm buccolingually, or a vertical mobility) (Miller 1950), Glickman advanced Grade II or Grade III/IV (through-and-through defect) furcation invasion (Glickman 1958), recalcitrant probing depth(s) greater than 8 mm, unfavorable crown-to-root ratio, and a history of recurrent periodontal abscesses. A tooth can also be extracted for aesthetic reasons or to improve the results of orthodontic treatment. When a surgical crown-lengthening procedure will lead to compromised esthetics, furcation invasion, and/or poor crown-to-root ratio, extraction is commonly advised (Becker et al. 1984, Chase and Low 1993).

Diagnosis

Diagnosis is a determination of any variations from what is considered normal. The dentist should be sensitive to the signs and symptoms presented and note any variations from normal. The dental diagnosis commonly includes a determination of the periodontal health, occlusal relationships, function of the temporomandibular joints (TMJs) and muscles of mastication, condition of edentulous areas, anatomic abnormalities, serviceability of existing prostheses and restorations, and status the of the remaining dentition.

TREATMENT-PLANNING PHASE

Sequencing of the treatment plan involves the process of scheduling the necessary procedures into a time-frame.

Effective sequencing is critical to the success of any treatment plan. Some treatment procedures must follow others in a logical order, while other treatment procedures can or must occur concurrently. Thus, thoughtful coordination is mandatory. Complex treatment plans are commonly sequenced into phases, including a control phase, an evaluative phase, a definitive phase, and a maintenance phase.

Control Phase

The control phase is divided into two parts: an initial periodontal phase and a provisional phase. This phase is intended to remove the etiologic factors, stabilize the patient's oral health, eliminate any active periodontal disease, and resolve inflammation. In this phase, often only a tentative treatment plan can be presented to the patient. Changes commonly occur relative to the prognosis of individual teeth at the termination of this phase. The initial periodontal phase includes extraction of hopeless teeth, periodontal debridement and scaling, oral hygiene instructions, and any indicated occlusal adjustments. The provisional phase then strives to remove conditions preventing effective maintenance, beginning the preventive dentistry component of the treatment. This phase includes caries control to determine restorability of teeth, replacement or repair of defective restorations, minor tooth changes, and an endodontic evaluation of all remaining teeth.

Evaluative Phase

The evaluative phase occurs between the control and the definitive phase. It allows for resolution of inflammation and time for healing. Home-care habits are reinforced, motivation for further treatment is assessed, and all preliminary treatment is reevaluated before definitive care is initiated.

Definitive Phase

After completing the control and the evaluative phase, the patient can enter the definitive phase. This phase begins with presenting the definitive treatment plan to the patient, including a wax replica of the proposed treatment plan. This phase is also divided into two parts: a preprosthetic phase and a prosthetic phase. The preprosthetic phase includes preprosthetic periodontal, oral surgical, endodontic, or orthodontic procedures. If implant surgery is proposed, then a computed tomographic (CT) scan is prescribed to evaluate the width and height of available bone as well as the location of vital structures, such as the inferior alveolar nerve, artery, and vein (inferior alveolar canal and mental foramen). The definitive phase is completed with the prosthetic phase for the fabrication and delivery of prostheses.

Some of the considerations and suggestions a dentist should follow when providing fixed prosthodontic treatment include the following (Morgano et al. 1989):

- A physiologic plane of occlusion
- A physiologic vertical dimension of occlusion (VDO)
- Simultaneous contacts of all anterior and posterior teeth in MIP
- A functional anterior guidance free of posterior interceptive occlusal contacts
- An unlocked arrangement of cusps and fossae that will allow comfortable jaw function
- Axial loading of posterior teeth
- The use of a material that will not unduly abrade the opposing dentition
- Narrowed occlusal tables, especially with implant-supported restorations, to minimize unfavorable leverage and bending moments

Maintenance Phase

This phase includes regular recall examinations that may reveal the need for adjustments to prevent future breakdown and provides an opportunity to reinforce home care. The frequency of this phase depends on the patient's risk for developing new dental disease. Maintenance visits are usually at 3- to 6-month intervals.

FINAL PROGNOSIS

The prognosis can be divided into a short- and long-term prediction, based on an educated forecast of the response to the planned treatment. It must take into account existing dental and periodontal support, vulnerability to expected disease, host resistance, the patient's adaptability, the dentist's capabilities, and expectations with regard to the patient's compliance with prescribed measures. When determining a prognosis, it should be tailored to the specific clinical situations. The prognosis can be (1) favorable, (2) guarded (questionable), (3) unfavorable (poor), or (4) hopeless. The dentist should provide a treatment plan that offers a favorable prognosis (McGuire 1991).

A *favorable prognosis* implies a high probability of success based on the best available evidence. A *guarded* or *questionable prognosis* suggests that one or more mitigating factors are present that are known to adversely affect the outcome of care. As an example, an endodontically treated tooth restored with a post-and-core and crown but lacking a ferrule would have a questionable prognosis (Morgano and Brackett 1999). An *unfavorable (poor) prognosis* implies a high probability of failure. A molar with a Glickman Grade III or IV furcation invasion will usually have a poor prognosis. Teeth with a *hopeless prognosis* cannot be treated with current materials and methods and must be extracted. An example is a pulpless tooth with a longitudinal root fracture that extends deeply into the alveolar bone.

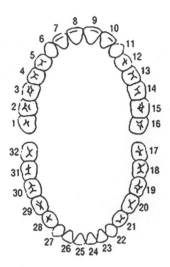

Fig. 6.1. Numbering system used in this chapter.

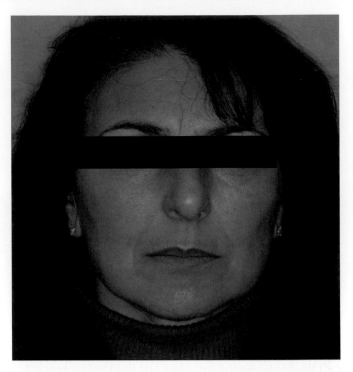

Fig. 6.2. Full-face frontal view of patient.

Patients

Throughout this chapter, the Universal Numbering System has been used to designate individual teeth. Figure 6.1 summarizes and illustrates this numbering system.

Patient I

A 43-year-old woman presented to the clinic with a chief complaint of, "I don't like my smile." (Figs. 6.2 and 6.3).

Diagnostic Phase

The patient's medical history was noncontributory. She did not have any known drug or food allergies. She did not smoke and drank alcohol only occasionally. Her dental history included orthodontic treatment that was performed many years previously to move the maxillary canines into the positions of the lateral incisors. She brushed twice per day and did not use dental floss. Extraoral examination revealed no cervical or submandibular lymphadenopathy and no signs of temporomandibular disorders (TMD) or reports of muscle pain.

The intraoral and radiographic examinations noted the following (Figs. 6.4 and 6.5):

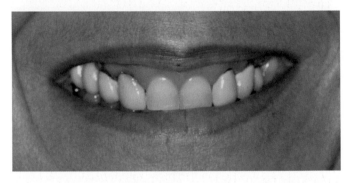

Fig. 6.3. Smile line.

- Missing Nos. 1, 5, 16, 17, and 32 and congenitally missing Nos. 7, 10, 20, and 19

- Maxillary canines in the position of the lateral incisors and restored with metal-ceramic crowns to mimic lateral incisors

- MO silver amalgam restorations, Nos. 2, 15, 30, and 31

- Metal-ceramic fixed partial dentures (FPDs), Nos. 3-x-5-6, and splinted crowns, Nos. 12-13-14

- MOD silver amalgam restoration, No. 16

- Defective MO silver amalgam restoration, No. 18

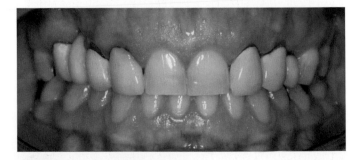

Fig. 6.4. Intraoral view.

- DO silver amalgam restoration, No. 20

- Occlusal silver amalgam restoration, No. 30

- Generalized inflammation with supragingival calculus in the mandibular anterior

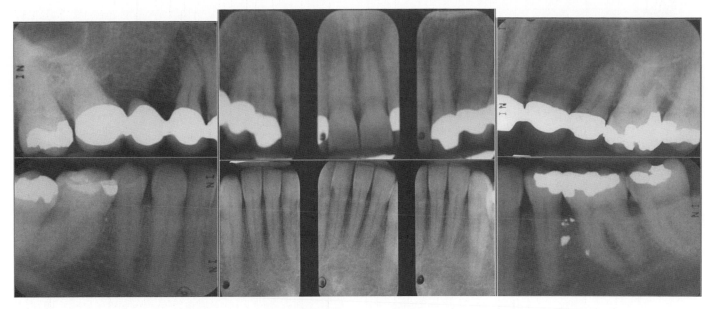

Fig. 6.5. Complete-mouth radiographs.

- Bony defect, site No. 4 (extraction site)

- Probing depths within normal range for most teeth with the exception of teeth No. 3 (distal 5 mm) and No. 14 (distal 5 mm) (Fig. 6.6)

- Rotated tooth, No. 12

- Absence of hypermobility or furcation invasion

The diagnosis for this patient was as follows:

- Generalized chronic mild gingivitis

- Localized chronic moderate periodontitis

- Partial edentulism

- Multiple defective dental restorations

Treatment Planning Phases

The objectives of therapy for this patient were elimination of the etiologic factors (open margins and defective restorations), control and resolution of periodontal inflammation, and restoration of esthetics and function. Initially, only a tentative treatment plan was presented to the patient. This plan in-

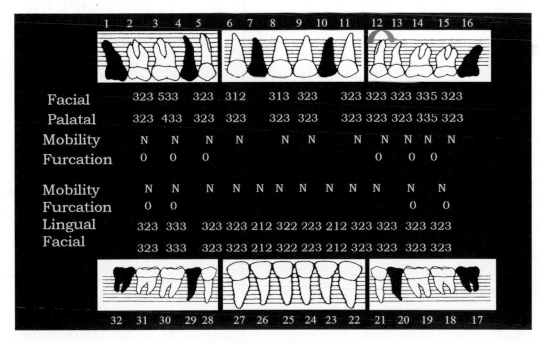

Fig. 6.6. Periodontal charting.

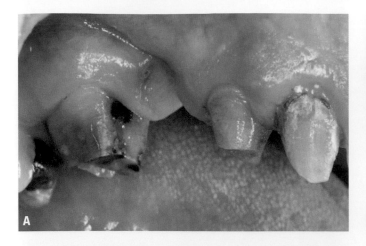

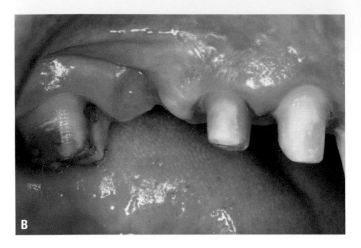

Fig. 6.7. A, Teeth Nos. 3, 5, and 6 after removal of defective restorations. **B,** Teeth after repreparation.

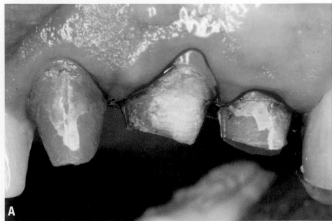

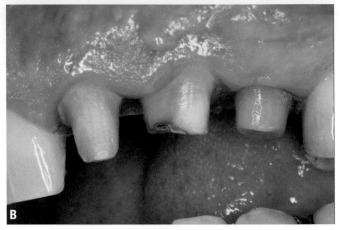

Fig. 6.8. A, Teeth Nos. 11, 12, and 13 after removal of defective restorations. **B,** Teeth after repreparation.

cluded the removal of artificial crowns, evaluation of the restorability of teeth, and plaque control measures.

Initial Periodontal Phase

This phase included scaling and root planing on the distal surfaces of Nos. 3 and 14, oral hygiene instructions, and reevaluation of any pocket reduction and oral hygiene.

Provisional Phase

In the provisional phase, the defective fixed restorations were removed (Figs. 6.7 and 6.8) and replaced with physiologically and aesthetically acceptable provisional restorations.

In evaluating the gingival line in the maxillae, a gingival line discrepancy was noted that was caused by the pontic in the area of No. 4. This discrepancy compromised the overall aesthetic

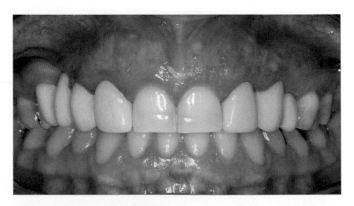

Fig. 6.9. Provisional restorations, Nos. 3-x-5, 6, 11, 12, and 13. Note the gingival line discrepancies at sites Nos. 3-x-5, 8-9, and 11-12-13.

appearance and contributed to plaque accumulation. There was also a gingival line discrepancy between the central incisors and the lateral incisors because the lateral incisors were originally canines that were orthodontically repositioned.

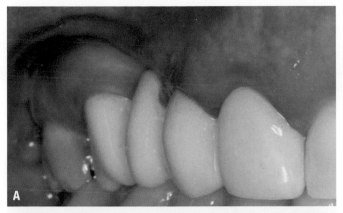

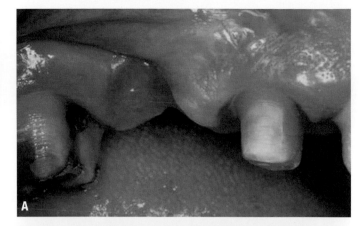

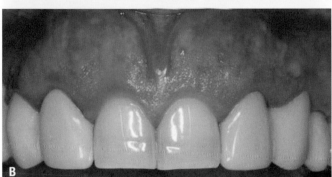

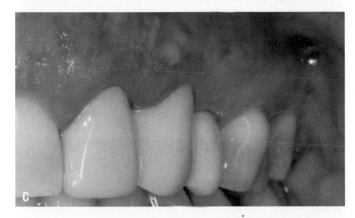

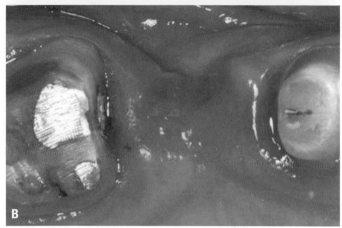

Fig. 6.11. **A, B,** Soft tissue inlay graft site No. 4, preoperative view.

Fig. 6.10. Preprosthetic treatment plan: **A,** Soft tissue augmentation, area No. 4. **B,** Microsurgical crown-lengthening procedure, Nos. 8 and 9, for aesthetic purposes. **C,** Crown-lengthening procedure, No. 13, for aesthetic purposes.

In addition, there was a gingival line discrepancy between Nos. 11, 12, and 13 (Fig. 6.9). Based on these findings, a definitive treatment plan was presented to the patient. This plan was (Fig. 6.10) as follows:

- Soft tissue augmentation, area No. 4

- Microsurgical crown lengthening procedure, Nos. 8 and 9 for aesthetic purposes

- Surgical crown-lengthening procedure, No. 13 for aesthetic purposes

- Metal-ceramic FPD, No. 3-x-5

- Ceramic crowns, Nos. 6 and 11

- Porcelain laminate veneers, Nos. 8 and 9

- Metal-ceramic crowns, Nos. 12 and 13

Preprosthetic Periodontal Phase

Soft tissue inlay graft, site No. 4. A split-thickness flap was elevated. Soft tissue augmentation for site No. 4 was accomplished by using an autogenous connective tissue inlay graft obtained from the patient's palate. The graft was sutured and secured to the periosteum. The flap was positioned and sutured without tension. The tissue surface of the pontic was relieved in the area of the surgical site to prevent tissue impingement. The pontic was relined 8 weeks after surgery with autopolymerizing acrylic resin (Coldpac; the Motloid Co., Chicago, IL, USA) to allow gentle pressure on the graft to contour the soft tissue at the pontic site and develop an esthetic gingival line. The pontic was relined again 1 week later to allow for additional contouring of the gingival line (Fig. 6.11).

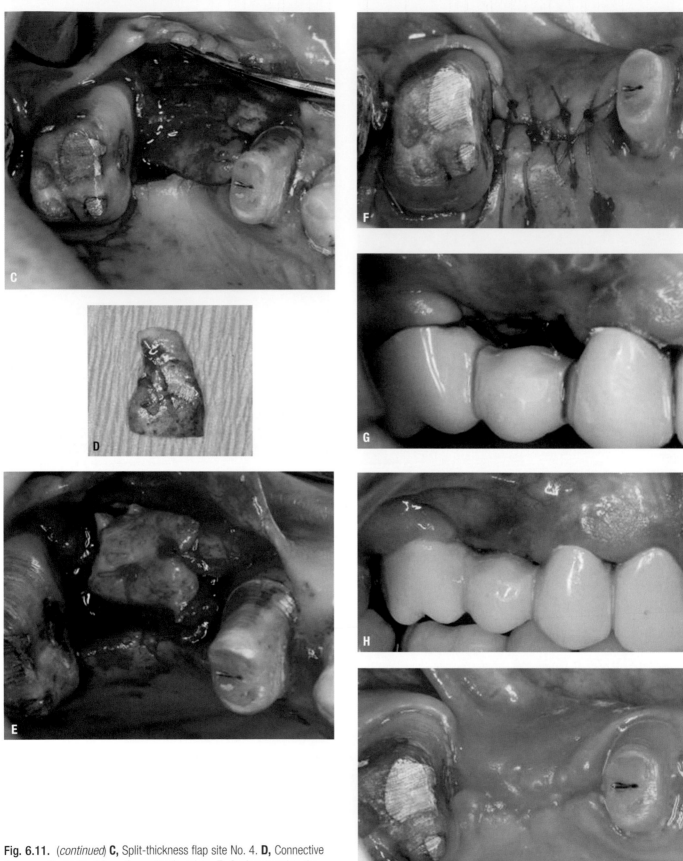

Fig. 6.11. (*continued*) **C,** Split-thickness flap site No. 4. **D,** Connective tissue graft obtained from the patient's palate. **E,** Graft sutured to the periosteum with chromic gut sutures. **F, G,** Flap sutured without tension. **H,** One week after surgery. **I,** Two months after surgery.

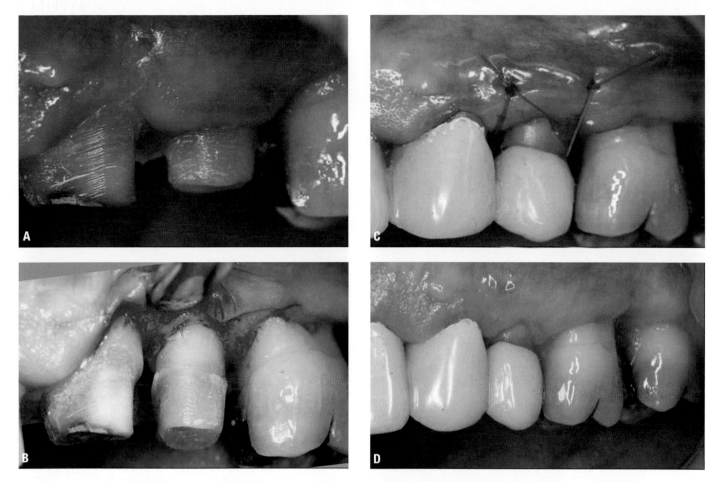

Fig. 6.12. Surgical crown lengthening procedure tooth No. 13. **A,** Preoperative view. **B,** 3-mm distance allowed between anticipated finish line of crown preparation and alveolar crest. **C,** Site sutured with vertical mattress technique and 4-0 chromic gut sutures. **D,** Two weeks after surgery.

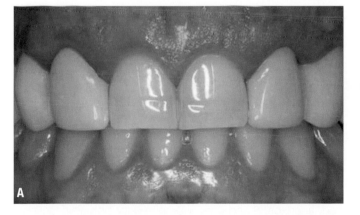
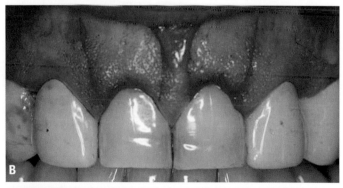

Fig. 6.13. Microsurgical crown-lengthening procedure for the facial surfaces of Nos. 8 and 9 to correct gingival line discrepancy. **A,** Preoperative view. **B,** Vertical incisions at the line angles of Nos. 8 and 9 by using a microsurgical blade.

Surgical crown lengthening, No. 13. A submarginal incision was made at the anticipated gingival line and a full-thickness flap was elevated. Ostectomy was performed to allow a 3-mm distance between the anticipated gingival line and the crest of the alveolar bone (Rosenberg et al. 1980).

The flap was repositioned and sutured with 4-0 chromic gut sutures (Fig. 6.12).

Surgical crown lengthening, Nos. 8 and 9. Surgical crown lengthening was required for aesthetic reasons on the facial surfaces of Nos. 8 and 9 only (Fig. 6.13).

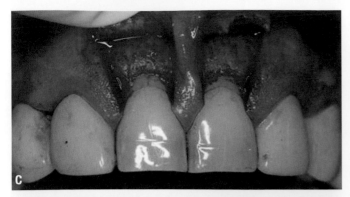

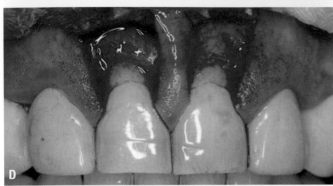

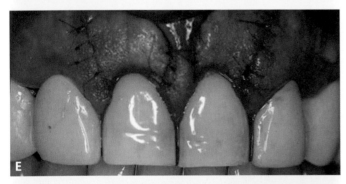

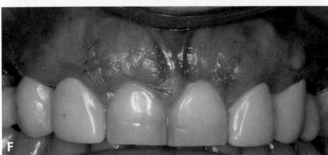

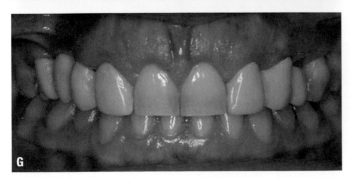

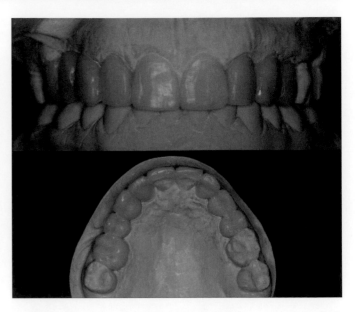

Fig. 6.14. Wax replica of proposed treatment plan.

To preserve the papillae and the soft tissue around Nos. 7 and 10, a microsurgical crown-lengthening procedure was performed. There are many advantages of this technique when compared with conventional surgical crown lengthening procedures (Dibart and Karima 2006). This procedure

- Is less invasive
- Requires smaller incisions
- Allows greater precision when closing wounds
- Is less traumatic
- Is less painful postoperatively
- Allows faster healing and vascularization
- Produces more predictable results in areas with very thin gingiva or in the "aesthetic zone"

Prosthetic Phase

Figure 6.14 is a wax replica of the proposed treatment plan.

Two months after completion of all periodontal surgical procedures, the margins for all crown preparations were finalized, and Nos. 8 and 9 were prepared for porcelain laminate veneers (Fig. 6.15).

New provisional restorations were fabricated, relined and cemented with temporary cement (Temp Bond; Kerr, Romulus, MI, USA) (Fig. 6.16).

Fig. 6.13. (*continued*) **C,** Full-thickness flap elevated. **D,** Ostectomy completed. **E,** Flaps sutured with 7-0 Vicryl sutures. **F,** One week after surgery. **G,** Two weeks after surgery.

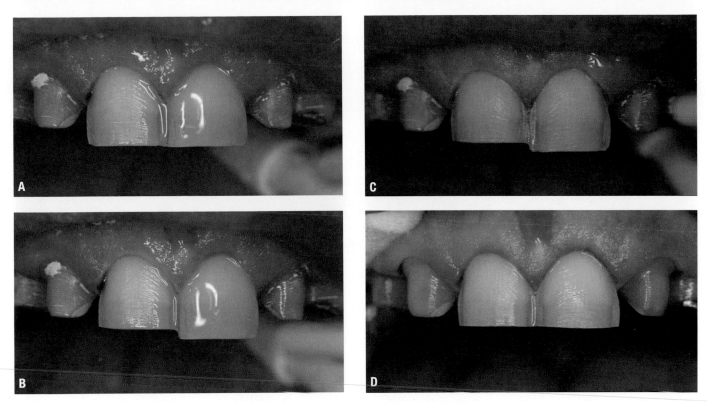

Fig. 6.15. Preparations for veneers, Nos. 8 and 9.

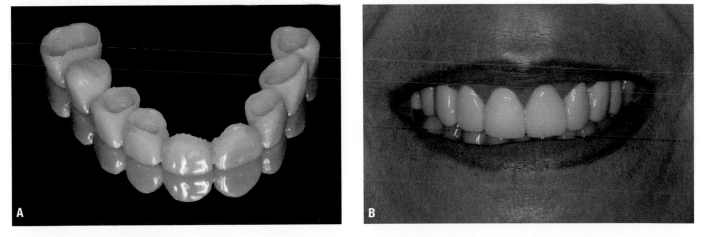

Fig. 6.16. Provisional restoration, Nos. 3-x-5-6-8-9-11-12-13. **A,** After contouring. **B,** In the mouth.

One week later, a final impression was made with polyether impression material (Permadyne Penta L and Impregum Penta; 3M ESPE, Seefeld, Germany) (Fig. 6.17).

A face-bow record was made and jaw relation records at MIP were made. A definitive cast was fabricated, along with a cast of the provisional restorations, and these casts were mounted in an articulator (Mark II Denar; Water Pik Technologies, Fort Collins, CO, USA). The shade was selected (Vita B1) (VITAPAN Classical Shade Guide; H Rauter GmbH & Co., Sackinggen, Germany). Porcelain laminate veneers for Nos. 8 and 9, zirconia copings for Nos. 6 and 11, metal copings for No. 12 and 13, and a metal framework for No. 3-x-5 were made. All copings and castings were tried in the mouth, and the fit was verified with black and white silicone disclosing material (Fit Checker; GC Corporation, Tokyo, Japan) (Fig. 6.18).

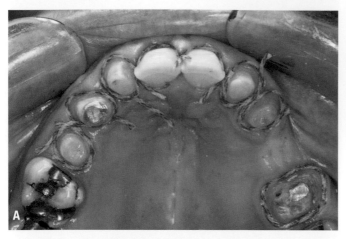
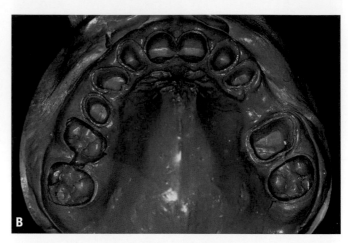

Fig. 6.17. A, Gingival displacement cord in place. **B,** Final impression with polyether impression material.

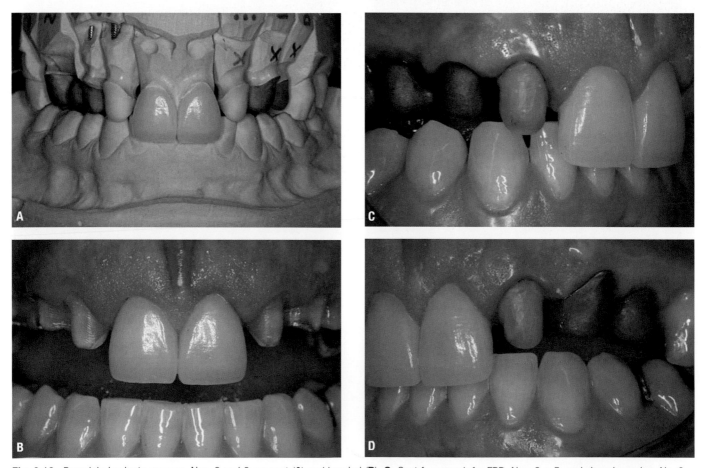

Fig. 6.18. Porcelain laminate veneers, Nos. 8 and 9, on cast (**A**) and bonded (**B**). **C,** Cast framework for FPD, Nos. 3-x-5, and zirconia coping, No. 6. **D,** Zirconia coping, No. 11, and castings for crowns, Nos. 12 and 13.

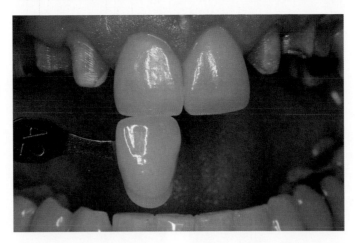

Fig. 6.19. Two weeks after cementation of veneers, shade was selected (Vita A2).

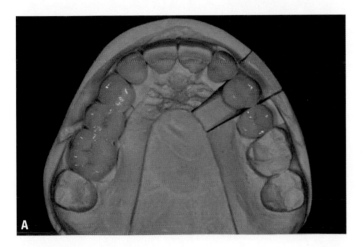

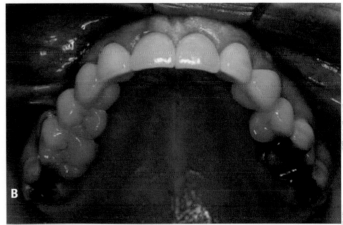

The veneers were luted with resin cement (Variolink II, Ivoclar Vitadent, Amherst, NY, USA). The provisional restorations for Nos. 3-x-5, 12, and 13 were recemented with Temp Bond cement. Because the resin luting agent requires an average of 2 weeks for the shade to mature beneath the veneers, the final shade selection for the remaining restorations was delayed. The final determination after 2 weeks was Vita A2 (Fig. 6.19).

At that stage, the application of porcelain to the remainder of the restorations was accomplished with Vita A2 porcelain. Restorations were glazed and the metal was polished. At the day of final delivery, provisional restorations were removed. A cleaning solution (Cavidry; Parkell, Farmingdale, NY, USA) was applied to all preparations to remove any oily residue, and clinical try-in of all restorations was completed. A resin-modified glass ionomer cement (Rely-X Luting; 3M ESPE) was used for final cementation of all restorations (Figs. 6.20

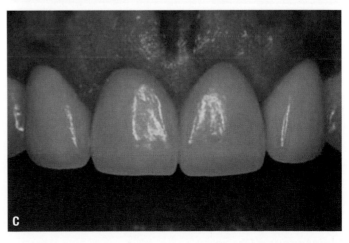

Fig. 6.20. A, Final restorations after porcelain application and glazing. **B,** Intraoral try-in. **C,** Corrected soft tissue profile Nos. 6, 8, 9, and 11.

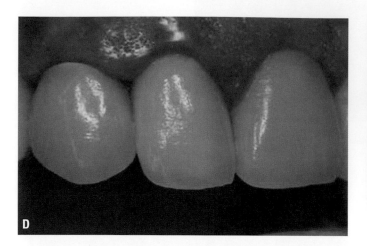

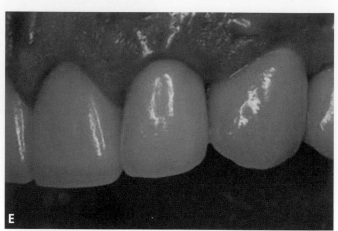

Fig. 6.20. (*continued*) **D, E,** All-ceramic crowns Nos. 6 and 11 with the clinical appearance of missing Nos. 7 and 10.

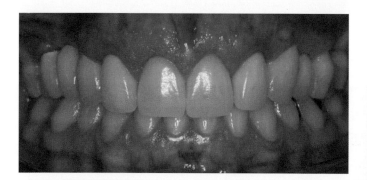

Fig. 6.21. Intraoral view of final restorations

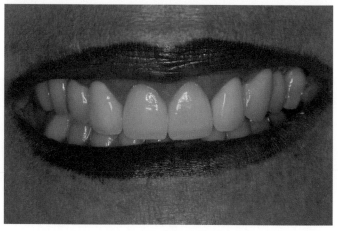

Fig. 6.22. Postoperative view of the new smile line.

to 6.23) 2 months after completion of all periodontal surgical procedures.

Maintenance Phase

The maintenance phase included recall visits every 4 months.

Prognosis

The overall prognosis for the treatment provided (short and long term) is favorable.

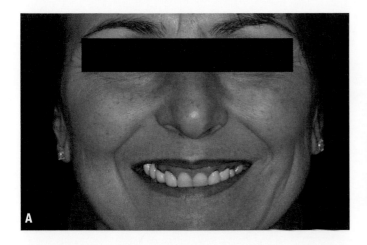

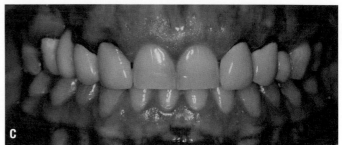

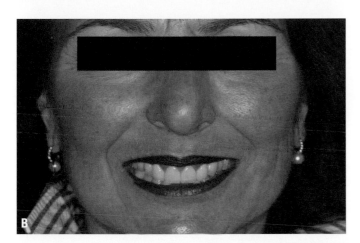

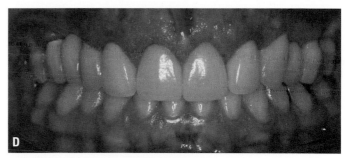

Fig. 6.23. Before (**A**) and after (**B**) (full-face view). Before (**C**) and after (**D**) (close-up view).

Patient II

A 70-year-old man presented to the clinic with a chief complaint of, "I need some implants for my lower jaw. My other dentist just finished all my upper teeth last year, and he sent me to you for the implants" (Fig. 6.24).

Diagnostic Phase

The patient's medical history was noncontributory. He did not have any known drug or food allergies. He had a previous history of smoking for 30 years, but for the past 3 years he has been using a nicotine patch and nicotine supplement gum. He had been smoke-free since then. He drank alcohol occasionally. His dental history included multiple extractions and fixed restorations. Extra-oral examination revealed no cervical or submandibular lymphadenopathy and no signs of TMD or reports of muscle pain.

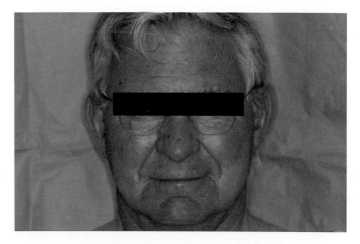

Fig. 6.24. Full-face frontal view of patient.

The intraoral and radiographic examinations revealed the following (Figs. 6.25 and 6.26):

- Missing, Nos. 1, 2, 3, 5, 14, 15, 16, 17, 19, 21, 23, 24, 25, 26, 29, 30, and 32
- Metal-ceramic FPD, Nos. 4-x-6
- Metal-ceramic crowns, Nos. 7, 8, 9, 10, 11, 12, and 13
- Defective metal-ceramic FPD, 22-x-x-x-x-27-28
- MOD silver amalgam restorations, Nos. 18 and 31
- Inadequate endodontic therapy, No. 20 with defective restoration
- Normal probing depths (between 2-3 mm), without bleeding upon probing, except for No. 18 where the probing depths were 6 mm on the mesial surface and 5 mm on the distal surface
- No hypermobility of the teeth or furcation invasions, except for No. 18, which had Class II hypermobility and Grade III furcation invasion

Maxillary and mandibular alginate impressions were made, along with a face-bow transfer and centric jaw relation record. The diagnostic casts were mounted in a semiadjustable articulator.

The diagnosis for this patient was as follows:

- Generalized mild gingivitis with localized moderate periodontitis, No. 18
- Partial edentulism
- Recurrent dental caries
- Defective dental restorations
- Inadequate endodontic treatment

Treatment Planning Phases

The treatment plan for this patient included the following:

- Extraction of Nos. 18, 20 and 31
- Implant-supported metal-ceramic crowns, sites Nos. 19-20-21 (immediate implant placement for No. 20), and 29
- Replacement of the defective metal-ceramic FPD, Nos. 22-x-x-x-x-27-28, to restore aesthetics and function

Initial Periodontal Phase

The initial periodontal phase included complete-mouth prophylaxis and oral hygiene instructions.

Preprosthetic Periodontal Phase

For the preprosthetic periodontal phase, a CT scan was prescribed and the proposed implant sites (Nos. 19, 20, 21, and 29) were evaluated (Fig. 6.27).

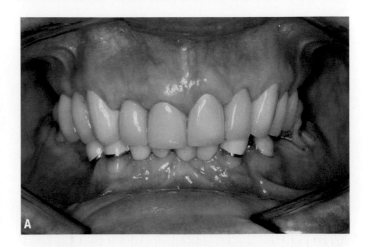
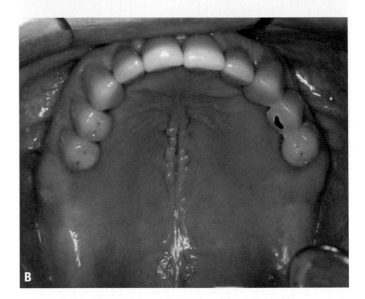
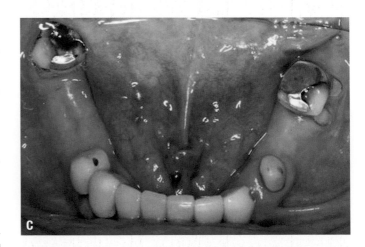

Fig. 6.25. Intraoral views. **A,** MIP. **B,** Maxillary arch. **C,** Mandibular arch.

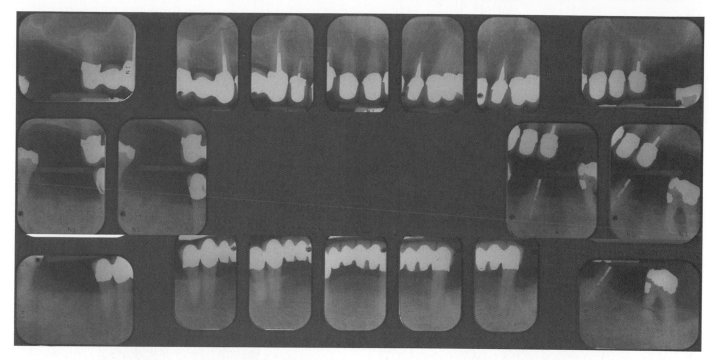

Fig. 6.26. Complete-mouth radiographs.

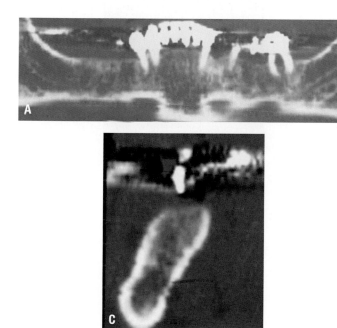

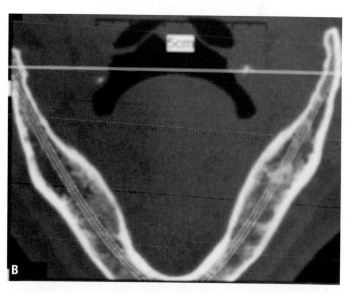

Fig. 6.27. CT scan evaluation. **A,** Panoramic cut. **B,** Horizontal cut. **C,** Segmental cut.

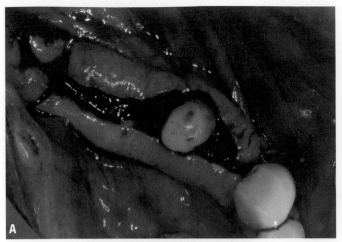

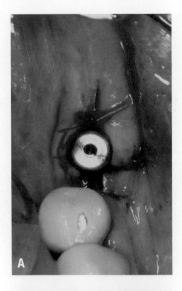

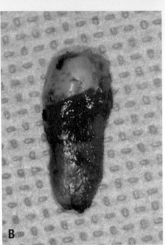

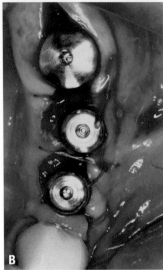

Fig. 6.29. Implants were uncovered 4 months later. **A,** Right side. **B,** Left side.

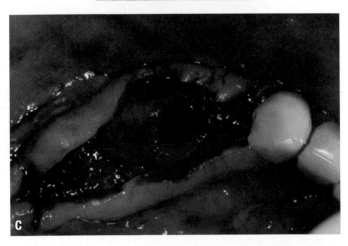

Fig. 6.28. Preprosthetic phase. Tooth No. 20 was extracted atraumatically. **A,** Incision. **B,** Extracted tooth. **C,** Undamaged socket (then implants were placed, Nos. 19, 20, 21, and 29).

Tooth No. 20 was extracted, and implants were placed at sites Nos. 19, 20 (immediate implant placement, No. 20), 21, and 29 (Fig. 6.28). Implants were uncovered 4 months after placement, and healing abutments were placed (Fig. 6.29).

Provisional Phase

The defective metal-ceramic FPD Nos. 22-x-x-x-x-27-28 was removed (Fig. 6.30).

After removal, it was discovered that No. 22 had a horizontal coronal fracture. Endodontic therapy was completed. A custom-cast post-and-core was made for No. 22 and cemented with zinc phosphate cement (Zinc Cement; Patterson Brand, Saint Paul, MN, USA) (Fig. 6.31).

An impression of the mandibular arch (implants Nos. 19, 20, 21, and 29 and all natural teeth) was made with polyether impression material (Permadyne Pental L and Impregum Penta) (Fig. 6.32).

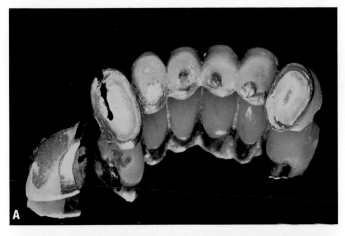

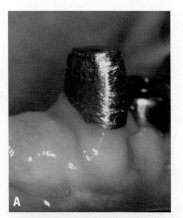

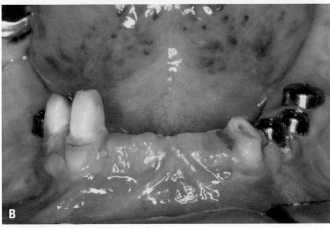

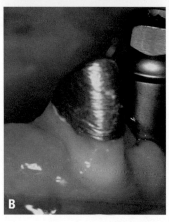

Fig. 6.31. Cast post-and-core. **A,** Try-in. **B,** Delivery.

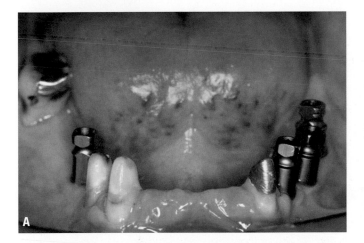

Fig. 6.30. A, Removal of defective FPD Nos. 22-x-x-x-x-27-28. **B,** Horizontal tooth fracture No. 22 was noted.

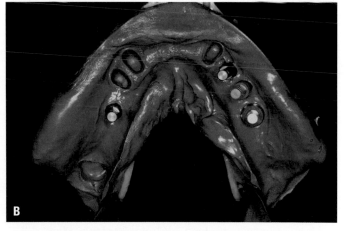

Fig. 6.32. Impression was made for fabrication of provisional restorations. **A,** Impression copings in place. **B,** Impression.

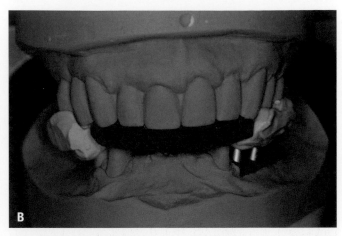
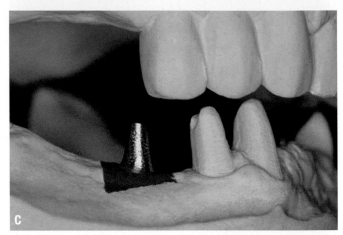

Fig. 6.33. A, Face-bow transfer. **B,** Casts mounted in centric relation.

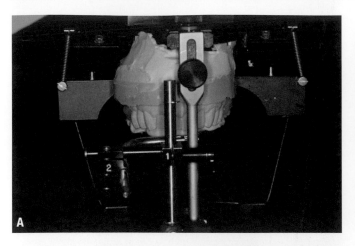
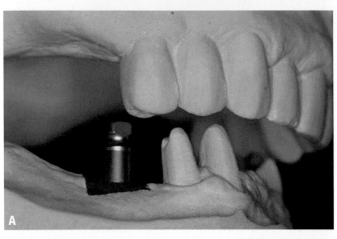
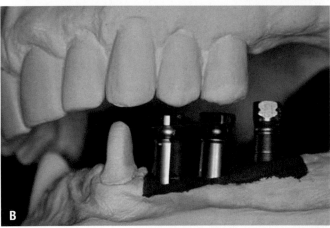
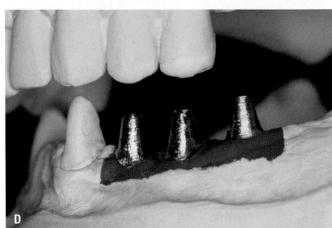

Fig. 6.34. Surgical mounts (**A, B**) of the dental implants were prepared to be used as temporary abutments (**C, D**).

Alginate impression material (Jeltrate; Dentsply, Melford, DE, USA) was used for the maxillary arch. A face-bow transfer was made, and a centric jaw relation record was made for the fabrication of the provisional restorations (Fig. 6.33).

The surgical mounts for the dental implants were prepared to be used as provisional abutments (Fig. 6.34).

A wax replica of the proposed treatment plan was prepared, and the wax pattern was invested and heat processed to produce an acrylic resin (Namilon; Justi, Oxnard, CA, USA) provisional restoration (Fig. 6.35).

The provisional FPD was cemented with Temp Bond cement (Fig. 6.36).

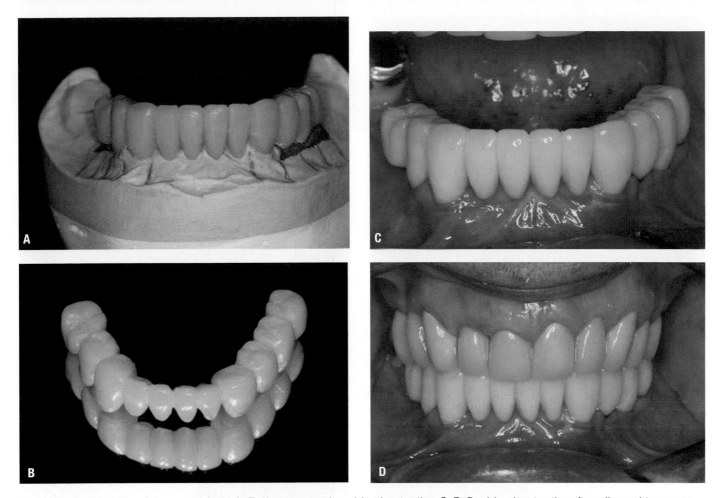

Fig. 6.35. A, Wax replica of the mandibular arch. **B,** Heat processed provisional restoration. **C, D,** Provisional restoration after reline and temporary cementation.

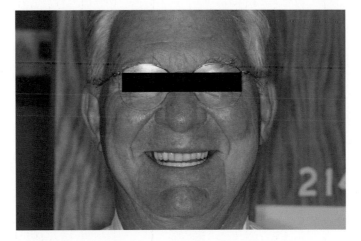

Fig. 6.36. Patient's smile after provisional restorations were placed.

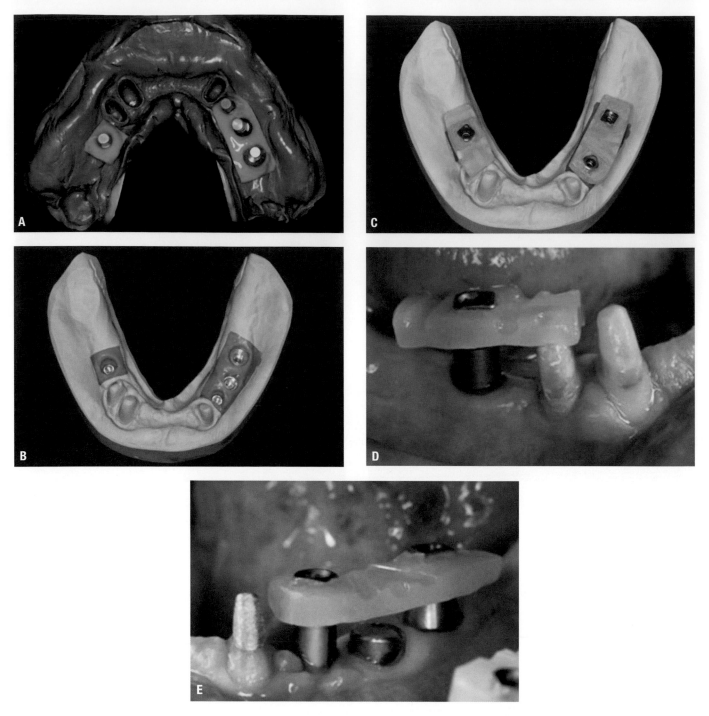

Fig. 6.37. A, Final impression made with polyether impression material. **B,** Soft tissue replicas around implant analogs. **C,D, E,** Fixed bilateral mandibular record bases for centric relation record.

Prosthetic Phase

Two weeks later, the patient presented for definitive impressions with polyether impression material (Permadyne Pental L and Impregum Penta) (Fig. 6.37).

A centric jaw relation record was completed and the mandibular cast was mounted. An alginate impression (Jeltrate) of the mandibular provisional restorations was made for the dental laboratory technician to use as a guide in the fabrication of the final restorations (Fig. 6.38).

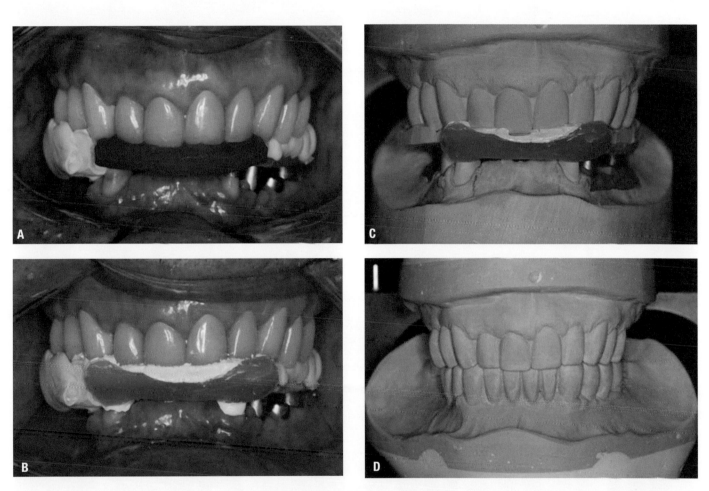

Fig. 6.38. **A,** Jaw relation record at centric relation with Lucia jig (Lucia, 1983) on anterior teeth and silicone registration material (Blu Mousse) on the posterior teeth. **B,** Lucia jig was then replaced with hard wax and relined with Temp Bond cement for stability of the casts during the mounting. **C,** Casts mounted. **D,** Diagnostic cast of existing mandibular provisional restoration was also mounted.

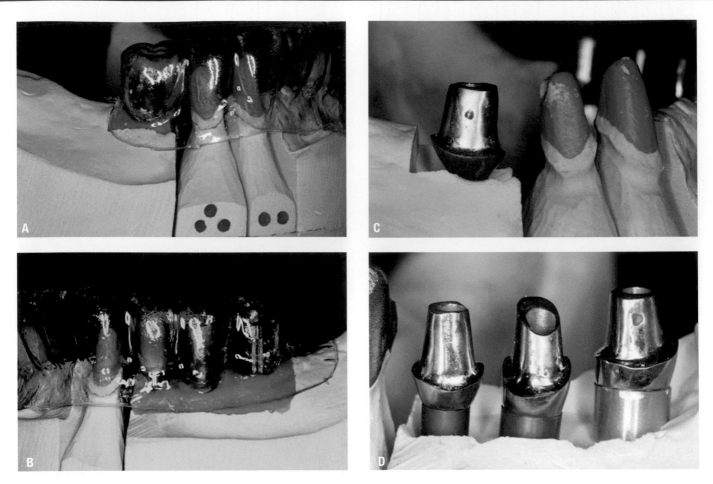

Fig. 6.39. A, B, Clear vacuum-formed shell of duplicate cast of patient's provisional restoration to be used as a three-dimensional guide for fabrication of custom abutments. **C, D,** Milled custom abutments.

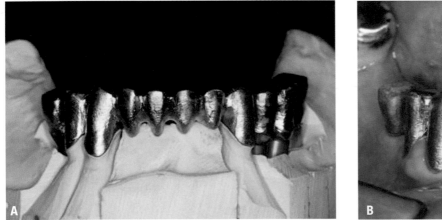
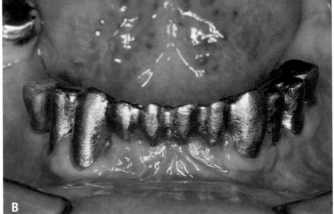

Fig. 6.40. A, Metal castings and frameworks. **B,** Metal try-in.

A clear plastic, vacuum-formed shell of the mandibular provisional restoration was also provided to the dental laboratory technician as a three-dimensional guide for the fabrication of the custom abutments (Fig. 6.39).

Metal castings and frameworks were fabricated. The fit of all metal castings was verified with silicone disclosing material (Fit Checker). The selected shade was Vita A2 (Fig. 6.40).

Metal castings and frameworks were returned to the dental laboratory for porcelain application (Fig. 6.41). Canine guid-

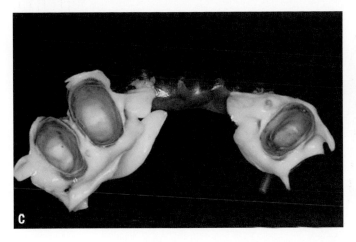

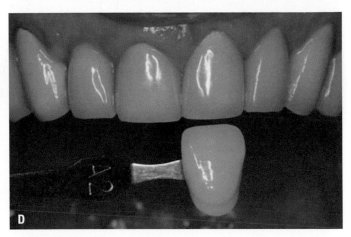

Fig. 6.40. (continued) **C,** Fit Checker silicone disclosing material to verify fit. **D,** Final shade was Vita A2.

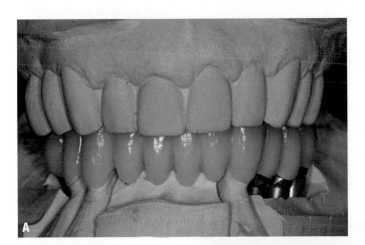

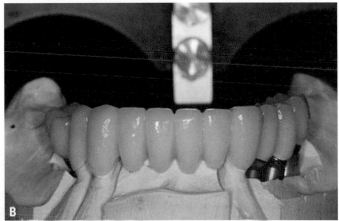

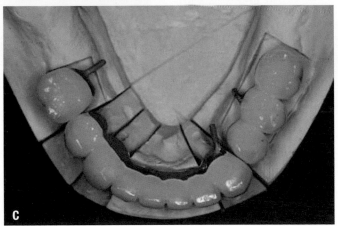

Fig. 6.41. Restorations after porcelain application. **A,** In occlusion. **B,** Frontal view. **C,** Occlusal view.

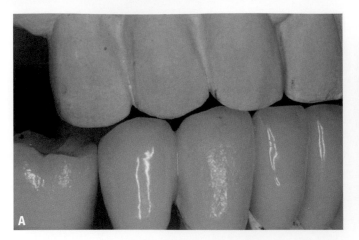
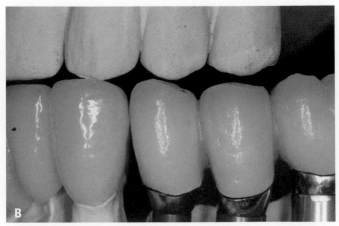

Fig. 6.42. Canine guidance. **A,** Right side. **B,** Left side.

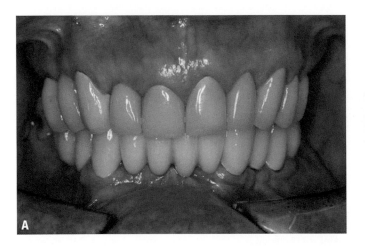
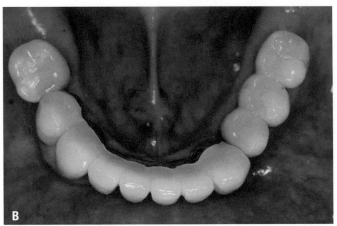

Fig. 6.43. Clinical try-in (**A**) and final delivery (**B**).

ance was established for the dynamic occlusal scheme (Fig. 6.42). Final delivery of the fixed prostheses was completed by using zinc phosphate cement (Zinc Cement) for the cementation of the tooth-supported FPD and by using Temp Bond cement for the cementation of implant-supported restorations (Figs. 6.43 to 6.45).

Maintenance Phase

The maintenance phase included recall visits every 3 to 4 months.

Prognosis

The overall prognosis for the treatment provided (short- and long-term) is favorable.

Patient III

A 40-year-old woman presented to the clinic with a chief complaint of, "I need new crowns, and I want a better smile" (Fig. 6.46).

Diagnostic Phase

The patient's medical history was noncontributory. She did not have any known drug or food allergies. She did not smoke or drink alcohol. Her dental history included multiple extractions and multiple restorations performed outside of the United States in 2001. She brushed twice per day and did not use dental floss. Extraoral examination revealed no cervical or submandibular lymphadenopathy and no signs of TMD or reports of muscle pain.

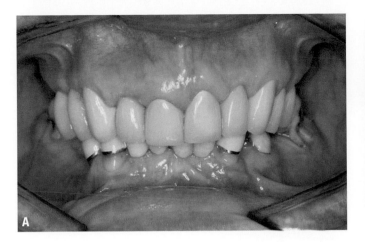

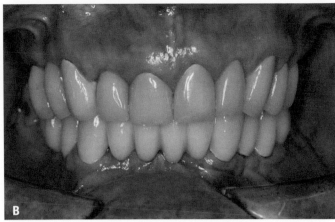

Fig. 6.44. Intraoral view before (**A**) and after (**B**) treatment.

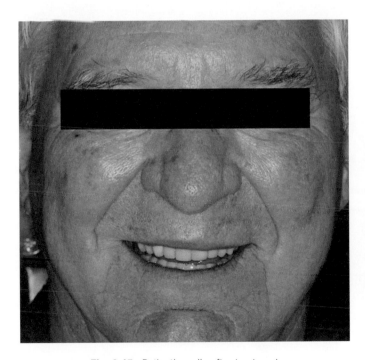

Fig. 6.45. Patient's smile after treatment.

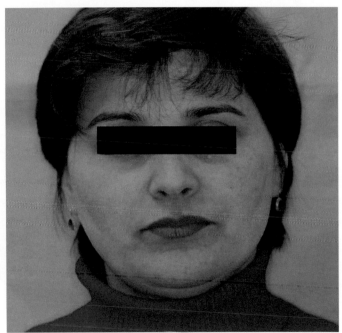

Fig. 6.46. Full-face frontal view of patient.

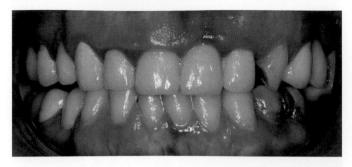

Fig. 6.47. Intraoral view.

The intraoral and radiographic examinations noted the following (Figs. 6.47 and 6.48):

- Generalized redness, edema, and glazing of the gingiva, especially in the maxillary anterior sextant

- Missing, Nos. 1, 3, 5, 9, 13, 14, 17, 18, 19, 28, 30, and 32

- Multiple defective restorations, Nos. 2-x-4-x-6, Nos. 7-8-x-10, and Nos. x-29-x-31

- Endodontic therapy, Nos. 4, 7, 11, 29, and 31

- Periapical radiolucency, No. 29

- Inadequate endodontic therapy, No. 31

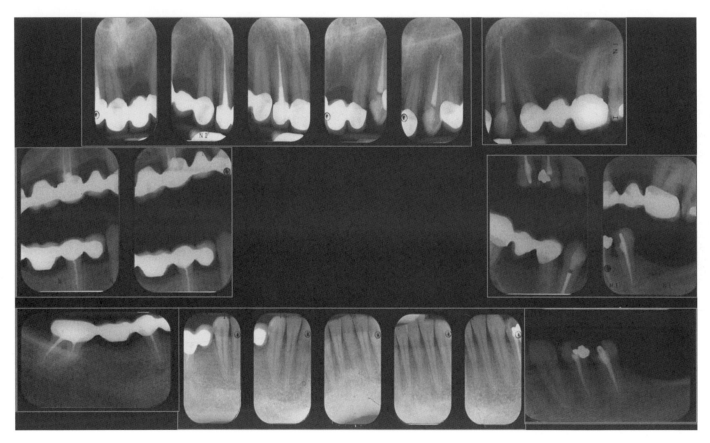

Fig. 6.48. Complete-mouth radiographs.

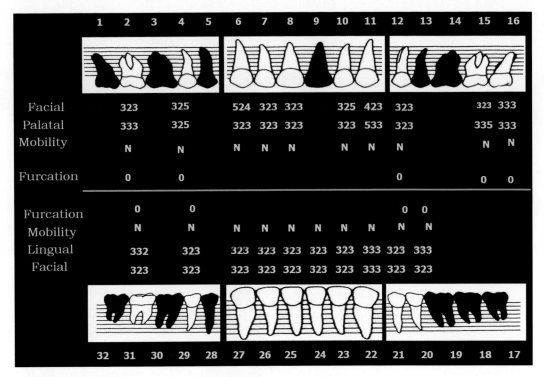

Fig. 6.49. Periodontal charting.

- Occlusal silver amalgam restoration, No. 16 with mesial and distobuccal carious lesions

- Mesial drift, Nos. 15 and 16

- Defective restorations, dental caries, and inadequate endodontic therapy, No. 20 and 21

- Distal carious lesions, Nos. 22 and 27

- Probing depths within the normal range (2 to 3 mm), except for teeth Nos. 4, 6, 10, 11, and 15, where probing depths ranged between 4 and 5 mm (Fig. 6.49)

- Generalized bleeding upon probing

- No hypermobility or furcation invasions (Fig. 6.49)

- Multiple defective FPDs

- Multiple teeth with inadequate endodontic therapy

- Localized bone loss (10% to 15%), distal surface of No. 15 and the mesial surface of No. 10 (Fig. 6.48)

Impressions were made with alginate (Jeltrate). Her diagnostic casts were mounted in centric relation in a semiadjustable articulator with a face-bow record (Fig. 6.50).

The diagnosis for this patient was as follows:

- Generalized moderate chronic gingivitis

- Localized moderate chronic periodontitis, No. 15

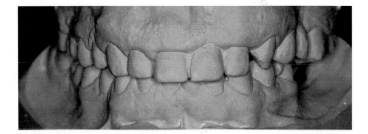

Fig. 6.50. Diagnostic casts.

- Partial edentulism

- Defective dental restorations

- Carious lesions

- Chronic periradicular periodontitis, No. 29

The etiologic factors contributing to this diagnosis were bacterial plaque as the primary factor and previous dentistry and patient neglect as secondary factors.

Treatment-Planning Phase

The objectives of therapy for this patient were elimination of the etiologic factors (open margins, overcontoured artificial crowns, inadequate endodontic therapy, and dental caries), control and resolution of periodontal inflammation, and restoration of aesthetics and function.

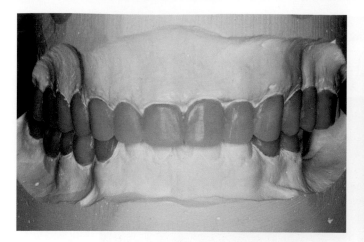

Fig. 6.51. Wax replica of tentative treatment plan.

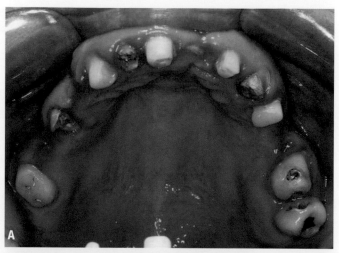

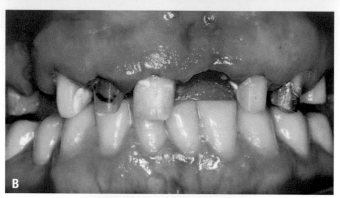

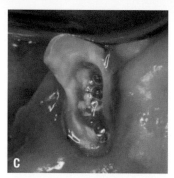

Fig. 6.52. A, B, Defective fixed restorations were removed. Note the compromised remaining tooth structure on No. 4 (**C**).

Initially, only a tentative treatment plan could be presented to the patient. This plan, according to the diagnostic waxing, included the following (Fig. 6.51):

- Removal of artificial crowns to evaluate the restorability of the teeth and to eliminate plaque retentive factors

- Extraction of No. 16

- Metal-ceramic FPDs, Nos. 2-x-4-x-6, 12-x-15, 27-x-29-x-31, and 8-x-10

- Metal-ceramic crowns, Nos. 7, 11, 20, and 21

- Endodontic retreatment, cast posts-and-cores, and metal-ceramic crowns, Nos. 7, 20, 21, 29, and 31

Initial Periodontal Phase

This phase included complete-mouth dental prophylaxis with scaling and root planning on the distal surface of No. 15, oral hygiene instructions, reevaluation of oral hygiene and pocket reduction, 3 to 4 weeks after the initial therapy.

Provisional Phase

The purpose of the provisional phase was the elimination of the etiologic factors and the maintenance of the health of the treated periodontium. The defective fixed restorations were removed and caries control was completed to evaluate the remaining teeth and determine their restorability and prognosis. At this stage, it was determined that all of her abutment teeth were restorable except for No. 4. Tooth No. 4 was compromised because of limited remaining tooth structure and deep subgingival margins (Fig. 6.52).

A crown-lengthening procedure would lead to furcation exposure and an unfavorable crown-to-root ratio. The recommended treatment was extraction of No. 4 and replacement with an implant-supported metal-ceramic crown. Caries con-

trol and temporization for teeth Nos. 20 and 21 were completed. Evaluation of the abutments indicated that surgical crown lengthening was required in the interproximal area between Nos. 20 and 21 (Fig. 6.53).

As a result of meticulous oral hygiene and replacement of the defective fixed restorations with physiologically and esthetically acceptable provisional restorations, the tissue health improved within 2 weeks, and the patient was satisfied with her appearance (Fig. 6.54). A gingival line discrepancy was noted between Nos. 8 and 9 (Fig. 6.55).

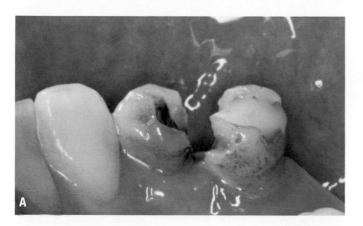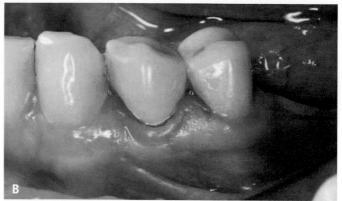

Fig. 6.53. Caries control and temporization, teeth Nos. 20 and 21. **A,** Facial view. **B,** Lingual view.

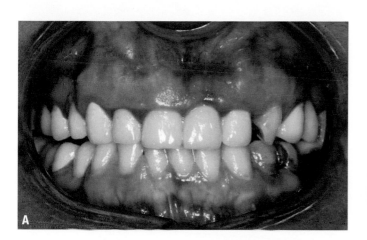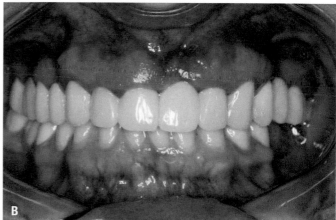

Fig. 6.54. Intraoral views before (**A**) and after (**B**) provisional restorations were placed. Note improved oral hygiene in **B.**

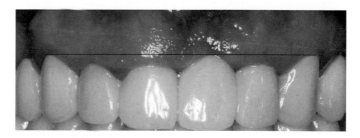

Fig. 6.55. Gingival line discrepancy.

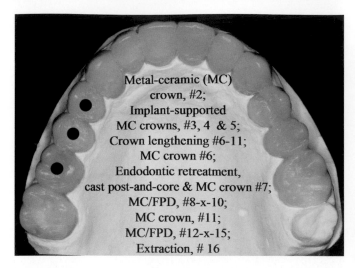

Fig. 6.56. Wax replica of finalized treatment plan for maxillary arch.

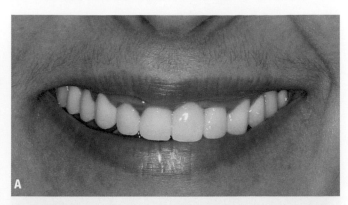

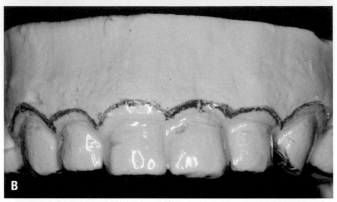

Fig. 6.58. Crown lengthening for the anterior sextant to gain crown length and for aesthetic purposes (**A**) with the use of a surgical guide template to assist the periodontist (**B**).

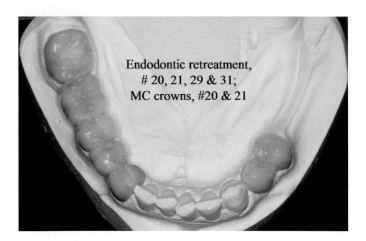

Fig. 6.57. Wax replica of finalized treatment plan for mandibular arch.

At this stage, the definitive treatment plan was presented to the patient (Figs. 6.56 and 6.57).

The treatment plan consisted of the following:

- Extraction of No. 16

- Metal-ceramic FPD, Nos. 8-x-10, 12-x-15

- Metal-ceramic crowns, Nos. 2, 6, 11, 20, 21, and 27

- Implant-supported metal-ceramic crowns, Nos. 3-4-5, 18-19, 28, and 31

- Surgical crown-lengthening procedure, Nos. 6 to 11

- Endodontic retreatment, cast posts-and-cores, and metal-ceramic crowns, Nos. 7, 20, 21, 29, and 31

The patient accepted the proposed treatment plan for the maxillae, but because of financial constraints, she accepted an alternative treatment plan for the mandible that included the following:

- Endodontic retreatment, Nos. 20, 21, 29, and 31

- Metal-ceramic crowns, Nos. 20 and 21

- Metal-ceramic FPD, Nos. 27-x-29-x-31

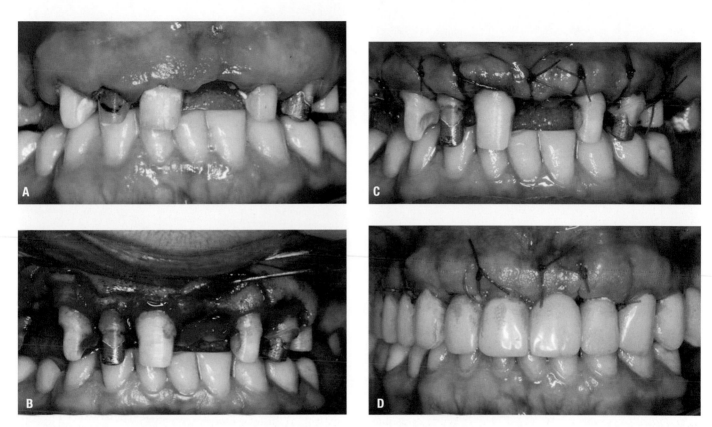

Fig. 6.59. Crown-lengthening procedure for teeth Nos. 6–11. **A,** Preoperative view. **B,** Full-thickness flap elevated and ostectomy performed. **C,** Closure with 4-0 chromic gut sutures. **D,** One week after surgery.

Preprosthetic Periodontal Phase

After the definitive treatment plan was presented to the patient, the patient entered phase III of the treatment, which was the pre-prosthetic periodontal phase. This phase began with surgical crown lengthening in the anterior sextant to obtain more crown length and to improve esthetics. A surgical guide was used (Fig. 6.58).

A full-thickness flap was elevated and ostectomy was performed to obtain a 3-mm distance between the anticipated gingival line Pas displayed in the template and the osseous crest, allowing space for the supracrestal gingival tissues. The flap was placed at the desired position and sutured with a vertical mattress technique by using 4-0 chromic gut sutures (Fig. 6.59).

After crown-lengthening procedures, a minimal healing period of 6 weeks was required before repreparation of the teeth and relining of the provisional restorations because 12 days are required for the junctional epithelium to form,

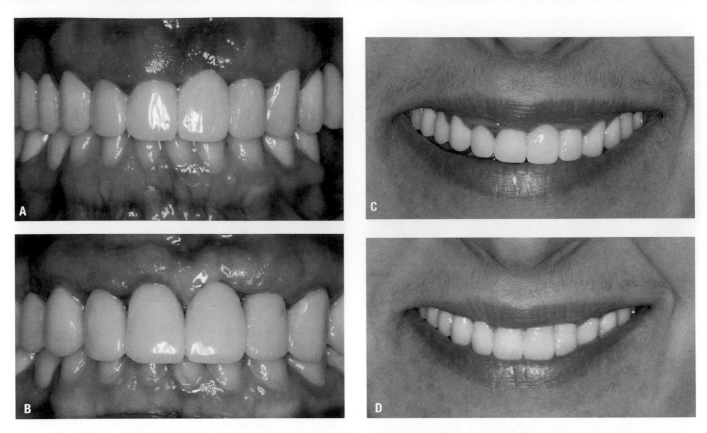

Fig. 6.60. Intraoral view before (A) and after (B) surgery. Smile before (C) and after (D) surgery.

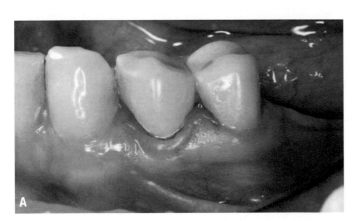

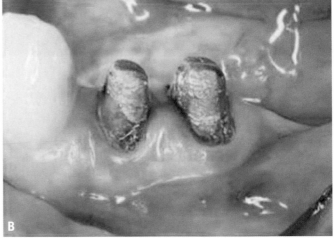

Fig. 6.61. Crown-lengthening procedure for teeth Nos. 20 and 21. A, Preoperative. B, Provisional crowns removed.

but the lamina propria is not completely formed until 6 weeks (Listgarten 1972) (Fig. 6.60). This patient also required a surgical crown lengthening procedure for Nos. 20 and 21. This procedure was required primarily in the interproximal area to ensure sufficient height of tooth structure to develop an acceptable ferrule effect. After flap elevation, ostectomy was completed, and the area was sutured with

a vertical mattress technique and 4-0 chromic gut sutures (Fig. 6.61).

The last phase of the preprosthetic periodontal phase was the implant phase for sites Nos. 3, 4, and 5. For this phase, the patient was referred for a CT scan with a dual-purpose template (Fig. 6.62).

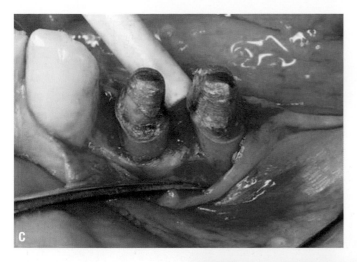

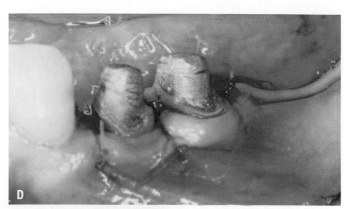

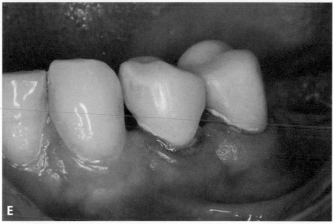

Fig. 6.61. (continued) **C,** Incision. **D,** Suturing. **E,** After suture removal.

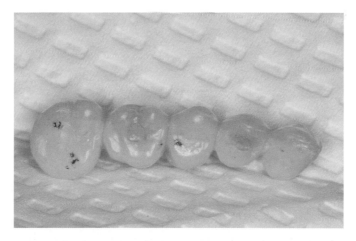

Fig. 6.62. Dual-purpose template for implants Nos. 3, 4, and 5.

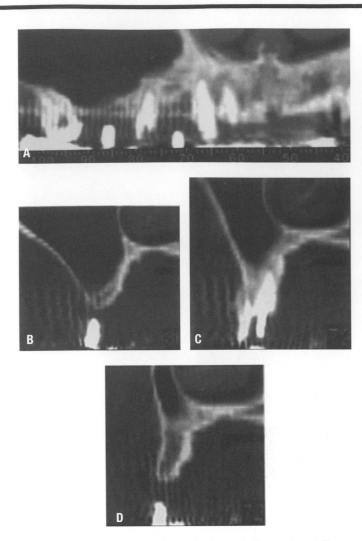

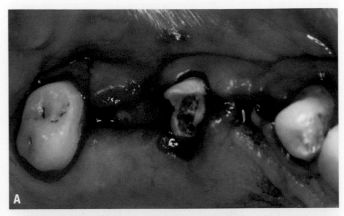

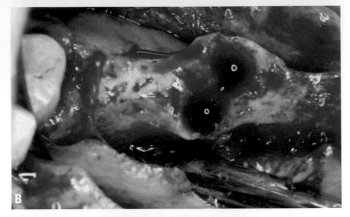

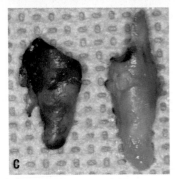

Fig. 6.63. CT scan evaluation for the implants. **A,** Panoramic cut. The segmental cuts. **B,** No. 3. **C,** No. 4. **D,** No. 5.

Fig. 6.64. Extraction of tooth No. 4. Note the Seibert's Class I ridge defect. **A,** Incision. **B,** Socket. **C,** Tooth sectioned and removed in two pieces.

The CT scan was evaluated for the selection of the size of the implants (Fig. 6.63).

For site No. 3, the available bone width was 5 mm and the height was 4 mm. The implant size planned for this site was 4 mm × 11.5 mm. Because of the location of the maxillary sinus and the width of the bone, the treatment plan for this site included a sinus floor elevation along with buccal augmentation of the residual alveolar bone with demineralized freeze-dried bone allograft (DFDBA; ACE Surgical, Brockton, MA, USA) and bovine bone (Bio-Oss; Osteohealth, Shirley, VA, USA).

For site No. 5, the available bone width was 5 mm and the height was 15 mm. The implant size planned for this site was 3.75 mm × 13 mm. Placing this implant according to the surgical guide would result in a thin buccal plate that is primarily composed of cortical bone; therefore, the recommended treatment included buccal augmentation with DFDBA (ACE surgical) and bovine bone (Bio-Oss).

A full-thickness flap was elevated, and tooth No. 4 was extracted. In evaluating the ridge at sites Nos. 3 and 5, Seibert's Class I ridge defect was noted (a defect in the buccolingual direction) (Seibert 1983) (Fig. 6.64).

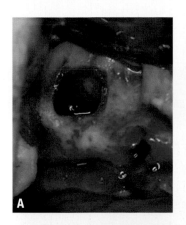

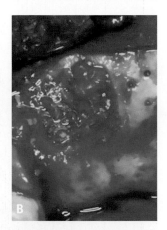

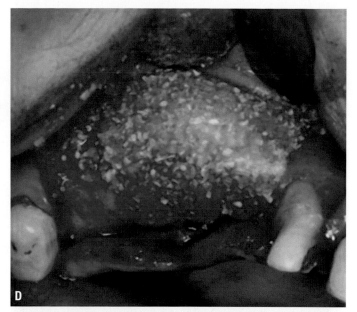

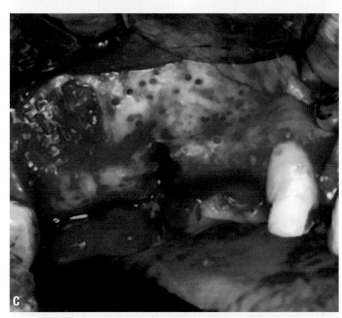

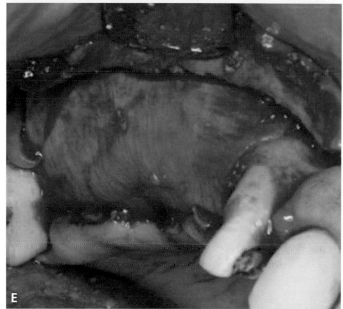

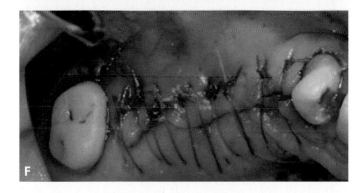

Fig. 6.65. Sinus floor elevation and guided bone regeneration. **A,** Lateral window approach performed and sinus membrane elevated. **B,** Sinus augmented with DFDB, Bio-Oss bovine bone, and autogenous bone. **C,** Decortication of buccal plate for ridge augmentation. **D,** Site grafted with DFDBA and Bio-Oss bovine bone. **E,** Resorbable membrane placed. **F,** Closure with 4-0 Vicryl sutures.

Sinus floor elevation for the site was accomplished by using the lateral window approach. The sinus membrane was elevated to receive an implant 11.5 mm in length. The sinus was grafted with DFDBA (Ace Surgical), bovine bone (Bio-Oss), and autogenous bone obtained from the palatal aspect of the surgical site. After the sinus was elevated and grafted, guided bone regeneration for sites Nos. 3, 4, and 5 was completed. The first step in accomplishing guided bone regeneration was decortication of the site with a No. 1 round carbide bur to increase the blood supply to the graft material. After decortication (Buser et al. 1990, 1996), the site was grafted with DFDBA (ACE surgical) and bovine bone (Bio-Oss). A resorbable membrane (Osteohealth) was used to protect and contain the graft material (Fig. 6.65).

The surgical area was closed without tension, and the pontic of the provisional FPD was trimmed away from the tissue to avoid irritation and facilitate plaque control. Another CT scan was made 9 months after surgery to determine the bone

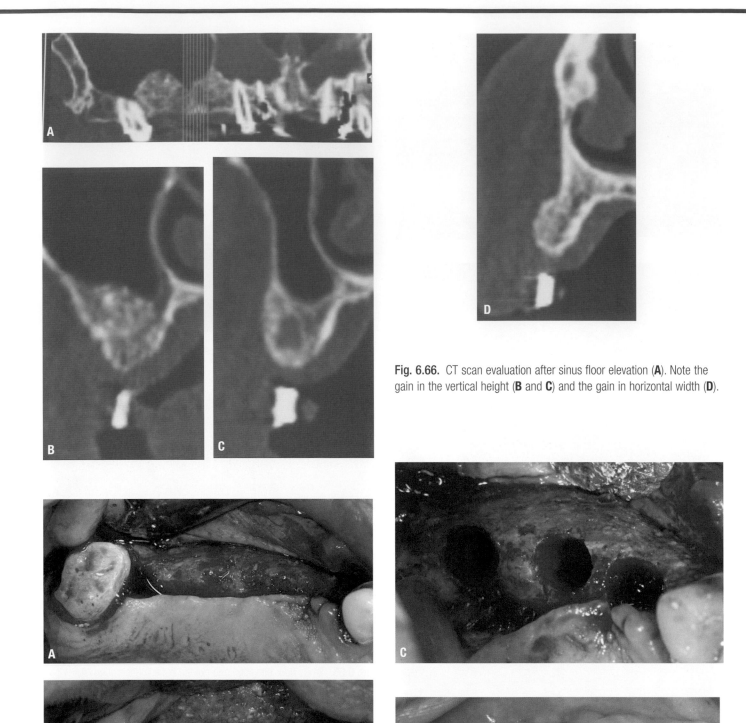

Fig. 6.66. CT scan evaluation after sinus floor elevation (**A**). Note the gain in the vertical height (**B** and **C**) and the gain in horizontal width (**D**).

Fig. 6.67. Implant placement sites Nos. 3, 4, and 5. **A,** Full-thickness flap elevated. **B,** The provisional restoration used as a surgical guide. **C,** Osteotomy sites. **D,** Implants placed.

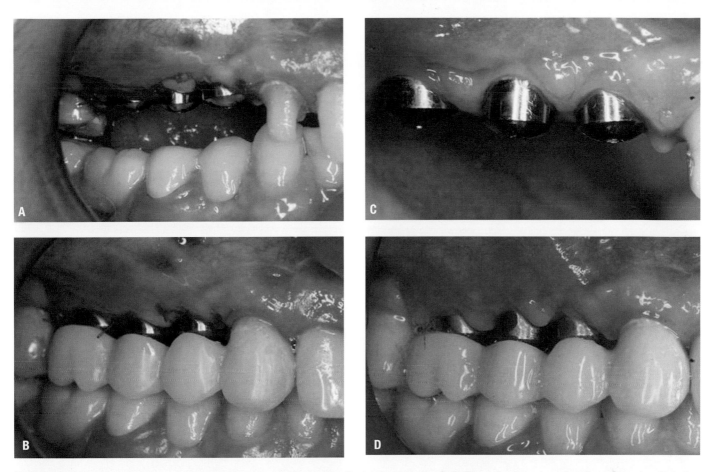

Fig. 6.68. Uncovering of implants. **A, B,** Implants uncovered 6 months after implant surgery. **C, D,** Tissue healing, 4 weeks after uncovering. Note formation of papillae.

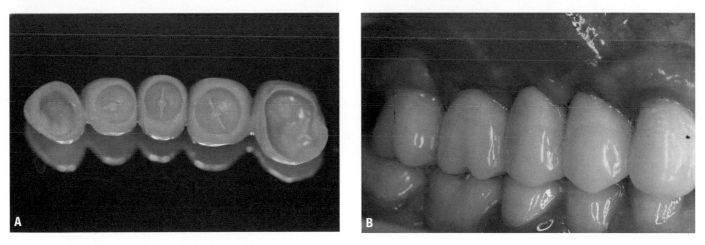

Fig. 6.69. Provisional restoration relined 4 weeks after uncovering. **A,** Intaglio surface. **B,** Provisional restoration in the mouth.

width and height in preparation for implant placement after the sinus elevation and grafting procedure (Fig. 6.66).

A full-thickness flap was elevated. The patient's provisional restoration was used as a surgical guide to place the implants. The flap was repositioned and sutured with 4-0 chromic gut sutures (Fig. 6.67).

Prosthetic Phase

The implants were uncovered six months after placement (Fig. 6.68). The provisional restoration was relined over the healing abutments 4 weeks after uncovering (Fig. 6.69).

Four weeks later, final impressions of all teeth and implants were made with polyether impression material (Permadyne

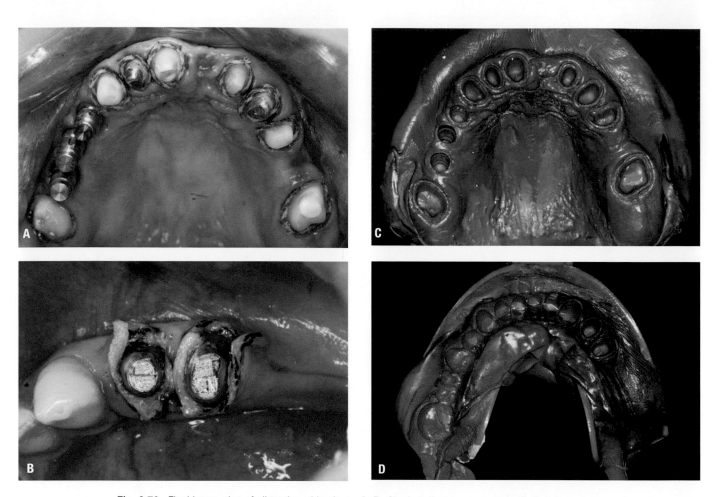

Fig. 6.70. Final impression of all teeth and implants. **A, B,** Gingival displacement cords. **C, D,** Impressions.

Penta L and Impregum Penta) and plastic stock trays (Coe Spacer Trays, Disposable Plastic Trays: GC America Inc., Alsip, IL, USA) (Fig. 6.70). A face-bow transfer and centric jaw relation record were made for the mounting of the definitive cast and for the cross mounting with the cast of the provisional restorations. A jig described by Lucia (Lucia 1983) was used as an anterior stop and extra-hard baseplate wax (Tru Wax; Dentsply, York, PA, USA) was used to make the record on the posterior teeth (Fig. 6.71). The definitive cast and the cast of the provisional restorations were mounted and cross-mounted (Fig. 6.72).

Die relief was placed on the dies (Die Spacer; Patterson Brand), and an artificial acrylic resin tooth (Pilkington Turner 30-degree tooth, 230 LS; Dentsply) was arranged to replace No. 19 at a height equal to half the height of the retromolar pad.

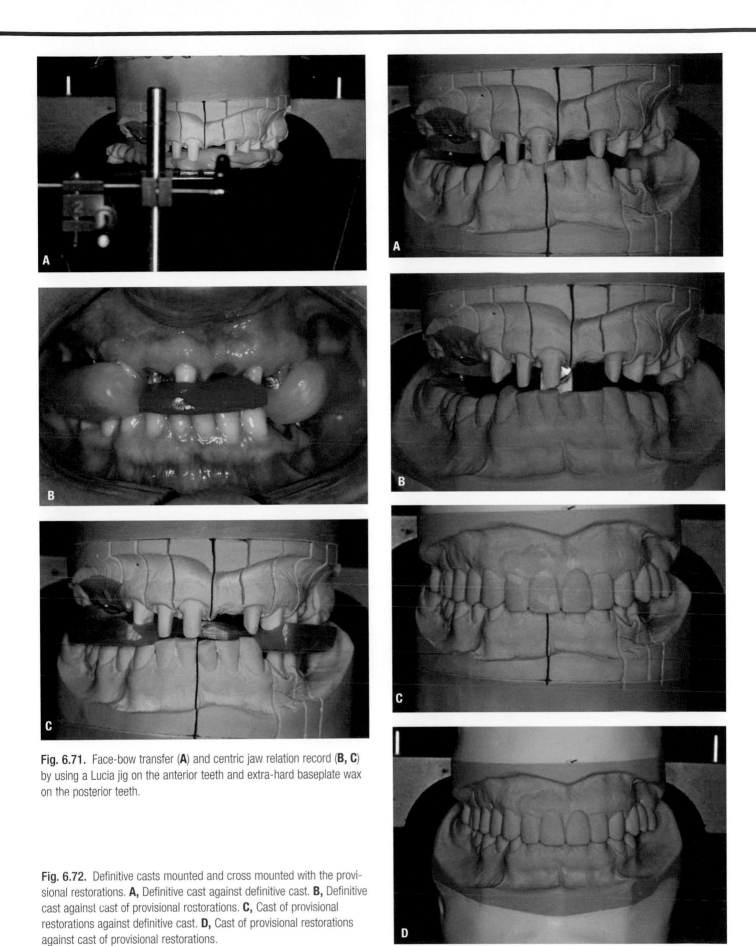

Fig. 6.71. Face-bow transfer (**A**) and centric jaw relation record (**B, C**) by using a Lucia jig on the anterior teeth and extra-hard baseplate wax on the posterior teeth.

Fig. 6.72. Definitive casts mounted and cross mounted with the provisional restorations. **A,** Definitive cast against definitive cast. **B,** Definitive cast against cast of provisional restorations. **C,** Cast of provisional restorations against definitive cast. **D,** Cast of provisional restorations against cast of provisional restorations.

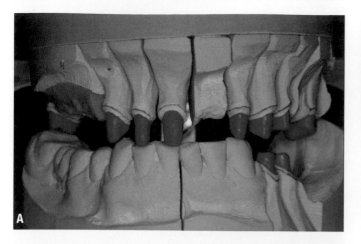

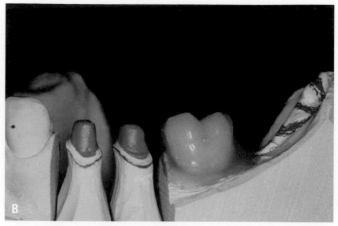

Fig. 6.73. **A,** Die relief placed on dies. **B,** Acrylic resin artificial tooth placed in position of No. 19 to establish occlusal plane at a height equal to half the height of the retromolar pad (marked in red).

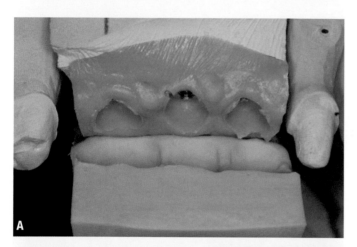

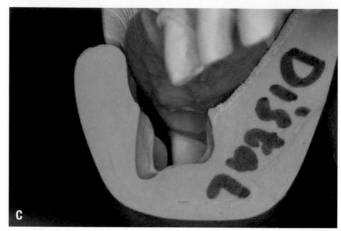

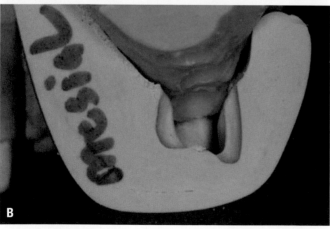

Fig. 6.74. Putty index of the provisional restoration was made to provide a three-dimensional view of the available space for custom abutments for implants. **A,** Facial view. **B, C,** Proximal views.

(Fig. 6.73). A putty (Exaflex Putty; GC America Inc.) index of the provisional restorations was made to provide a three-dimensional view of the available space to the dental laboratory technician for the fabrication of the custom abutments (Fig. 6.74).

A clinical try-in was accomplished to verify the position of the custom abutments by using a verification jig fabricated from light polymerizing urethane dimethacrylate resin (Triad Tru

Tray VLC Custom Impression Tray Material; Dentsply) on the definitive cast (Fig. 6.75). At try in, it was noted that the custom abutment for No. 4 was rotated on the cast. The verification jig was relieved in the area of No. 4, and autopolymerizing resin material (Pattern resin LS: GC America Inc.) was used to reline and re-register the position of the custom abutment in the mouth. This relationship was then transferred to the definitive cast by altering the cast (Fig. 6.76).

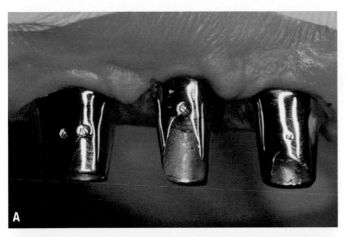

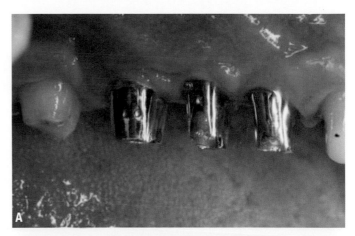

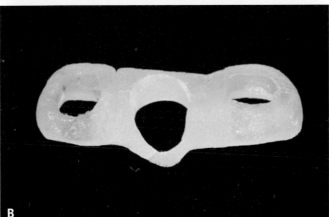

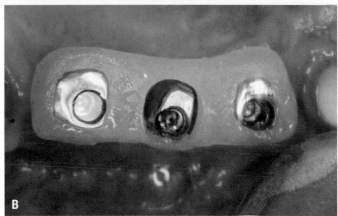

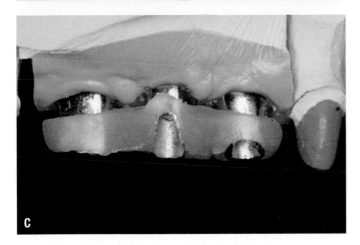

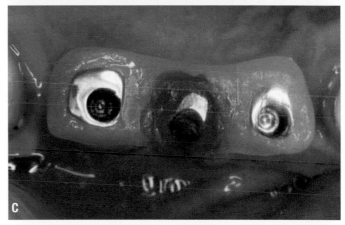

Fig. 6.75. A, Custom abutments were fabricated. **B, C,** Verification jig was made.

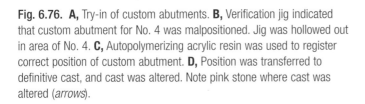

Fig. 6.76. A, Try-in of custom abutments. **B,** Verification jig indicated that custom abutment for No. 4 was malpositioned. Jig was hollowed out in area of No. 4. **C,** Autopolymerizing acrylic resin was used to register correct position of custom abutment. **D,** Position was transferred to definitive cast, and cast was altered. Note pink stone where cast was altered (*arrows*).

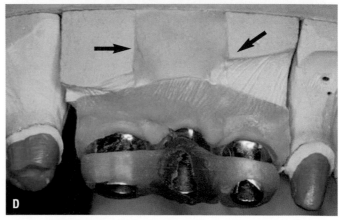

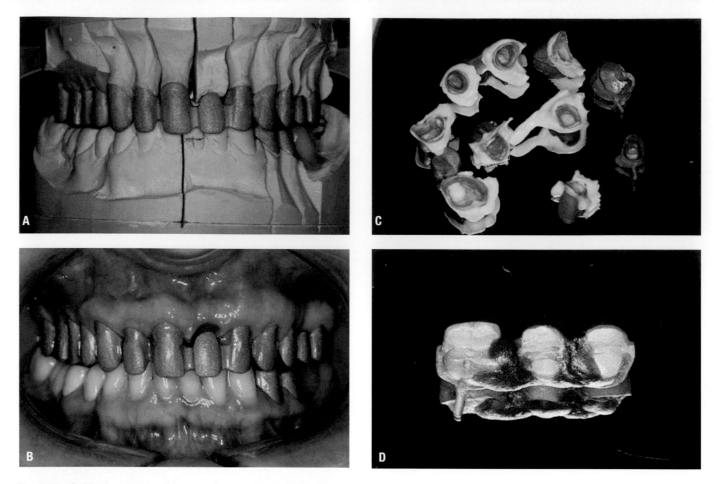

Fig. 6.77. A, Metal castings and frameworks were fabricated. **B,** Castings were tried in the mouth. **C,** Fit verified with silicone disclosing material (Fit Checker). **D,** Metal framework for implant-supported splinted crowns, Nos. 3–5, was sectioned, and reconnected with autopolymerizing acrylic resin in preparation for soldering.

Metal castings and frameworks were fabricated. The castings were tried in the mouth, and the fit was verified with a silicone disclosing material (Fit Checker). The framework was sectioned between Nos. 3-4 and 4-5 and then soldered (Fig. 6.77). The soldered casting for Nos. 3-4-5 was tried again in the mouth, and the fit was verified.

A second jaw relation record was made at the desired VDO with the use of a Lucia jig as an anterior stop and extra-hard baseplate wax (Tru Wax; Dentsply) on the posterior teeth. A pick-up impression was made of the metal castings with the use of polyether impression material (Permadyne Penta L and Impregum Penta). The casts were mounted and sent to the dental laboratory for porcelain application (Fig. 6.78). The shade selected was Vita B1, as per the patient's request.

At the porcelain bisque try-in, modifications to proximal and occlusal contacts were made. Some adjustments were made also to the contours of the restorations. Canine guidance was established. The restorations were then sent for final glazing. At the day of final delivery, gold screws for the custom abutments Nos. 3, 4, and 5 were torqued to 32 N•cm with a torque wrench (Torque Indicator; 3I, Palm Beach Gardens, FL, USA). The abutments were then torqued again to 32 N•cm after a 10-minute waiting period to compensate for embedment relaxation of the screws.

All restorations were cemented with Rely-X Luting resin-modified glass ionomer cement, with the exception of the implant-supported restorations Nos. 3-4-5, which were cemented with temporary cement (Temp Bond) after sealing the screw holes with a temporary sealer (Dura-Seal; Reliance, Worth, IL, USA). Temporary cement was used for the implant-supported restorations to ensure retrievability (Figs. 6.79 and 6.80).

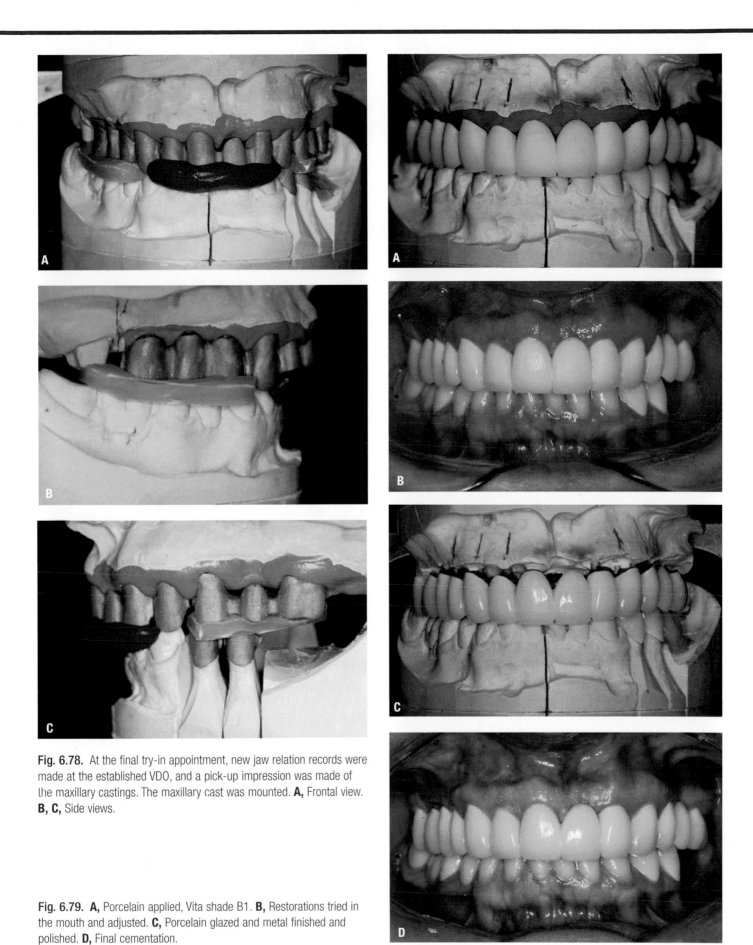

Fig. 6.78. At the final try-in appointment, new jaw relation records were made at the established VDO, and a pick-up impression was made of the maxillary castings. The maxillary cast was mounted. **A,** Frontal view. **B, C,** Side views.

Fig. 6.79. A, Porcelain applied, Vita shade B1. **B,** Restorations tried in the mouth and adjusted. **C,** Porcelain glazed and metal finished and polished. **D,** Final cementation.

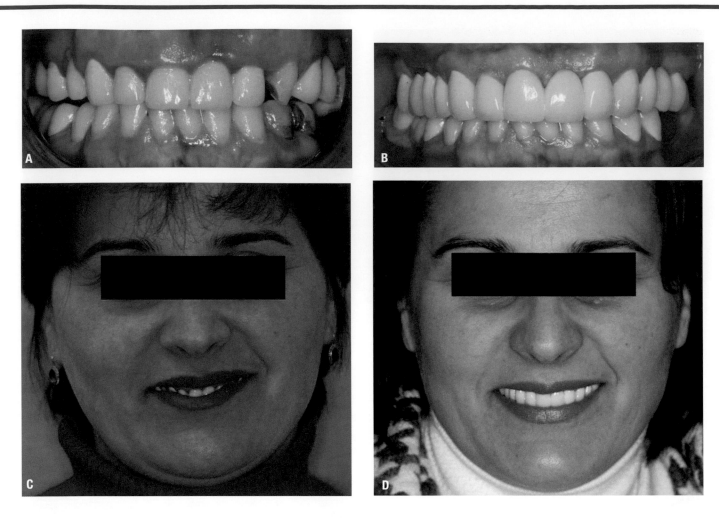

Fig. 6.80. Intraoral views before (**A**) and after (**B**). Smile before (**C**) and after (**D**).

Maintenance Phase

The maintenance phase included recall visits every 3 to 4 months.

Prognosis

The overall prognosis for the treatment provided (short and long term) is favorable.

CONCLUSION

The overall quality of dental care depends on a concerted effort among the various dentists involved, a thorough and complete diagnosis that addresses all disease processes, and a realistic, carefully sequenced treatment plan that offers a favorable prognosis.

REFERENCES

AAP position paper. Periodontal considerations in the management of cancer patients. Committee on Research, Science and Therapy of the American Academy of Periodontology. 1997. *J. Periodontol.* 68:791–801.

Becker, W., L. Berg, and B. Becker. 1984. The long-term evaluation of periodontal treatment and maintenance in 95 patients. *Int. J. Periodont. Restor. Dent.* 2:55–72.

Buser, D., U. Bragger, N.P. Lang, et al. 1990. Regeneration and enlargement of jaw bone using guided tissue regeneration. *Clin. Oral Implants Res.* 1:22–32.

Buser, D., K. Dula, H.P. Hirt, et al. 1996. Lateral ridge augmentation using autografts and barrier membranes: A clinical study with 40 partially edentulous patients. *J. Oral Maxillofac. Surg.* 54:420–432.

Chase, R., Jr., and S.B. Low. 1993. Survival characteristics of periodontally-involved teeth: a 40-year study. *J. Periodontol.* 64:701–705.

Davies, R. 1993. Antibiotic prophylaxis in dental practice. *Br. Med. J.* 307:1210–1211.

Dibart, S, and M. Karima. 2006. *Practical Periodontal Plastic Surgery.* Ames, IA, Blackwell Publishing.

Flocken, J.E. 1980. Electrosurgical management of soft tissues in restorative dentistry. *Dent. Clin. North Am.* 24:247–269.

Glickman, I. 1958. *Clinical Periodontology,* 2nd ed. Philadelphia, W.B. Saunders, pp. 694–696.

Listgarten, M.A. 1972. Normal development, structure, physiology and repair of gingival epithelium. *Oral Sci. Rev.* 1:3–67.

Listgarten, M.A. 1972. Ultrastructure of the dento-gingival junction after gingivectomy. *J. Periodont. Res.* 7:151–160.

Lucia, V.O. 1983. *Modern Gnathological Concepts—Updated.* Chicago, Quintessence, pp. 83–107.

McGuire, M. 1991. Prognosis versus actual outcome: a long-term survey of 100 treated periodontal patients under maintenance care. *J. Periodontol.* 62:51–58.

Mealey, B.L., and T.W. Oates. 2006. Diabetes mellitus and periodontal diseases. *J. Periodontol.* 77:1289–1303.

Miller, S.C. *Textbook of Periodontia,* 3rd ed. Philadelphia, Blackstone, 1950, p. 125.

Morgano, S.M., P.M. Garvin, B.L. Muzynski, and W.F. Malone. 1989. Diagnosis and treatment planning. In W.F. Malone, D.L. Koth, E. Cavazos Jr., D.A. Kaiser, and S.M. Morgano, editors. *Tylman's Theory and Practice of Fixed Prosthodontics,* 8th ed. St Louis, Ishiyaku EuroAmerica, pp. 1–23.

Morgano, S.M., and S.E. Brackett. 1999. Foundation restorations in fixed prosthodontics: current knowledge and future needs. *J. Prosthet. Dent.* 82:643–657.

Rosenberg, E.S., D.A. Garger, and C.I. Evian. 1980. Tooth lengthening procedures. *Compend. Cont. Educ. Dent.* 1:161–173.

Seibert, J. 1983. Reconstruction of deformed, partially edentulous ridges, using full thickness onlay grafts. Part I. Technique and wound healing. *Compend. Cont. Educ. Dent.* 4:437–453.

Soileau, K.M. 2006. Oral post-surgical complications following the administration of bisphosphonates given for osteopenia related to malignancy. *J. Periodontol.* 77:738–743.

Thomson, W.M., H.P. Lawrence, J.M. Broadbent, and R. Poulton 2006. The impact of xerostomia on oral-health-related quality of life among younger adults. *Health and quality of life outcomes.* 4:86 (published online before print November 8, 2006).

Wooltorton, E. 2005. Health and Drug Alerts: Patients receiving intravenous bisphosphonates should avoid invasive dental procedures. *Can. Med. Assoc. J.* 172:1684.

Chapter 7 The Contribution of Periodontics to the Correction of Vertical Alveolar Ridge Deficiencies

Serge Dibart, DMD

ALVEOLAR DISTRACTION OSTEOGENESIS SURGERY

History

Alveolar distraction surgery is an application of Ilizarov's distraction osteogenesis method to the maxillofacial skeleton. Between 1954 and 1971, Gavriel Ilizarov, a Russian orthopedic surgeon, developed a novel surgical approach for reconstruction of skeletal deformities. This involved the use of a mechanical device (the distractor) and the formation of new bone between the bone segments that were gradually separated by incremental traction (Birch and Samchukov 2004). This traction generated tension that stimulated new bone formation parallel to the vector of distraction (Cope and Samchukov 2001, Samchukov 1998). This technique had the added advantage of displacing and preserving the soft tissue with the mobilized bony segment. This is particularly useful in the process of alveolar distraction where the alveolar housing and the surrounding soft tissue are displaced together in a single, simultaneous process (Block 1996, Chin and Toth 1996, McCarthy 1995, Ortiz Monasterio 1997).

Indications

- Combined deficiencies in hard and soft tissue not allowing for dental implant placement

- Vertical alveolar ridge deficiency impairing the placement of a dental implant or fixed partial denture (Figs. 7.1 and 7.2)

- Axial correction of misaligned osseointegrated dental implants or ankylosed teeth

- Orthodontics: Therapy of local open bite

Limitations

- Must have a minimum of 6 mm of residual bone height

- Must have adequate bone width (otherwise block graft necessary before distraction)

- Thin residual bony arch, presenting the risk of fracture

- Patients on bisphosphonates

- Irradiated patients (>40 to 60 Gy)

- Malignancies

- Heavy tobacco use

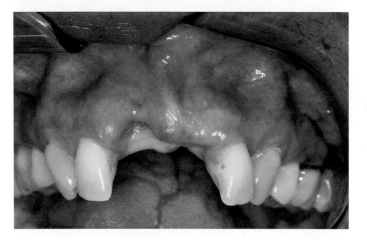

Fig. 7.1. Patient presenting with a vertical height defect subsequent to the loss of teeth Nos. 8 and 9.

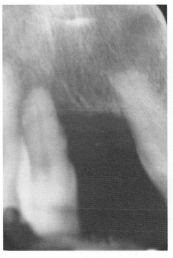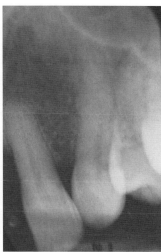

Fig. 7.2. Tooth No. 8 will be extracted due to severe periodontal disease. Notice the lack of vertical height of the alveolar bone.

Advantages (Chiapasco 2004)

- Eliminates the need to harvest bone

- Less operating time

- Distraction histogenesis

117

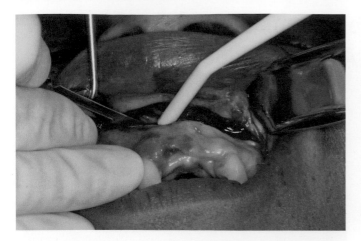

Fig. 7.3. The incision is high up in the vestibule to allow for flap mobilization and access.

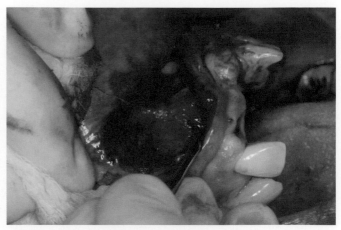

Fig. 7.4. The full-thickness flap is reflected using a periosteal elevator.

- Lower risk of morbidity of the surgical site
- Crestal part of the distracted segment has lower risk of resorption
- Greater vertical bone gain

Armamentarium

- Standard surgical kit, as described in *Practical Periodontal Plastic Surgery* plus:
- Alveolar Distraction Track Plus Kit (KLS Martin, Jacksonville, FL, USA) and oscillating and sagittal microsaws (KLS Martin, Jacksonville, FL, USA)

Technique for the Anterior Segment

After proper local anesthesia (infiltration with xylocaine 2% with 1:100,000 epinephrine and 1:50,000 epinephrine for hemostasis), an incision is made in the vestibule using a No. 15 blade. The incision is made high enough in the mucosa to allow for proper mobilization of the flap (Fig. 7.3). The incision may be done in two steps: incision of the mucosal layer first, then incision of the connective tissue, muscles, and periosteum. Keep the blade oriented toward the alveolar bone. The incision has to be long enough to allow for easy blunt dissection with a periosteal elevator.

The role of the elevator is to now reflect the flap all the way up to the alveolar crest of the edentulous site but not beyond (Figs. 7.4 and 7.5). It is critical to leave the palatal or lingual periosteum attached to the bone, because it will be the only source of vascularization of the bony fragment during the distraction process. Once the bony area is exposed, it is useful to draw a picture of the segment to be distracted on the bone using a sterile No. 2 pencil (Fig. 7.6). The base of the bony segment should be wider at the crest than apically (Fig. 7.7) to allow for unimpaired sliding movement during the traction

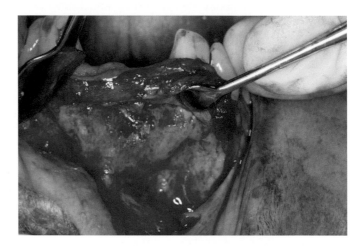

Fig. 7.5. Reflection stops at the alveolar crest.

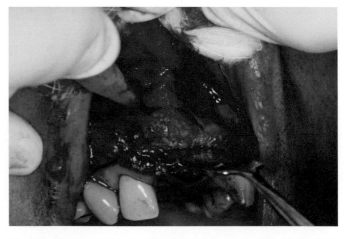

Fig. 7.6. The segment to be distracted is delineated with a sterile No. 2 pencil.

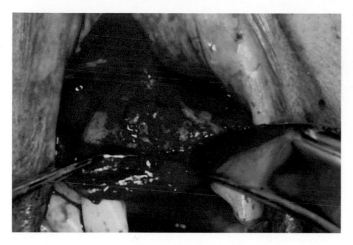

Fig. 7.7. The segment to be cut is drawn on the bone. Notice the divergence of the cuts that will allow for free movement of the segment.

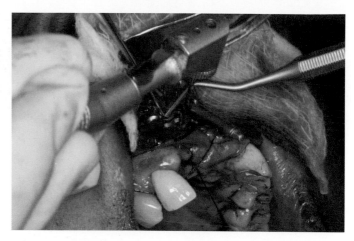

Fig. 7.10. One hole in each arm of the distractor is predrilled; this will allow accurate repositioning of the device.

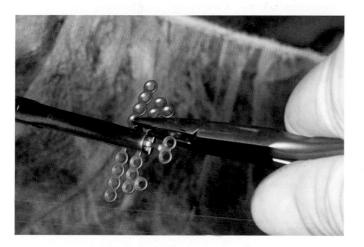

Fig. 7.8. The distractor is modified to fit the clinical picture.

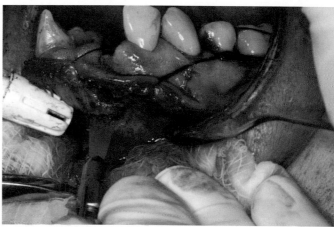

Fig. 7.11. Using the oscillating microsaw (KLS Martin, Jacksonville, Fl, USA), the osteotomy is started.

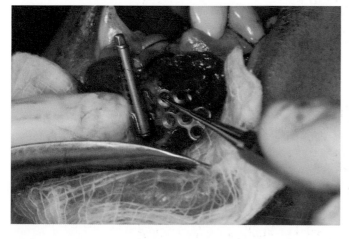

Fig. 7.9. The distractor is placed, verifying the correct direction of the distraction vector.

process. Also at this point, it is important to remember that the distracted segment should be no shorter than 5 mm.

Once the segment is visualized, it is time to adapt the distractor to fit the clinical picture. This is the most time-consuming part of the operation, because one has to adapt (cut) and bend the upper and lower arms of the distractor to fit the underlying bone architecture, while preserving the proper direction of the vector (Figs. 7.8 to 7.10). Distractors are available in 6-, 9-, 12-, and 15-mm lengths. After predrilling one hole for each arm while holding the distractor in place, the sagittal saw (set at 20,000 RPM) is used to cut the bone (Fig. 7.11). It is better not to do a through-and-through cut at the beginning but to get as close as possible to the palatal/lingual bony

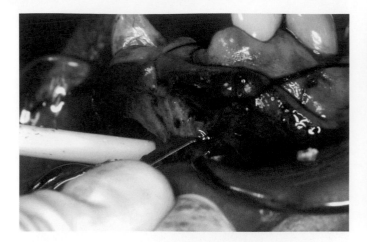

Fig. 7.12. It is important to get as close as possible to the palatal/lingual cortical plate but not go through it with the sagittal microsaw, so as not to injure the palatal/lingual periosteum.

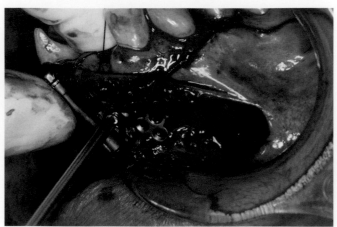

Fig. 7.14. The distractor is repositioned very accurately due to the previously drilled holes and secured with the screws.

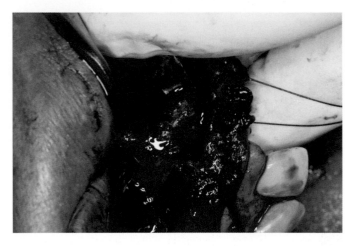

Fig. 7.13. A fine osseous chisel (or modified spatula) is used very carefully with a mallet in order to detach the segment to be distracted. Notice the finger on the palate; it is used to counteract and control the force of the blow.

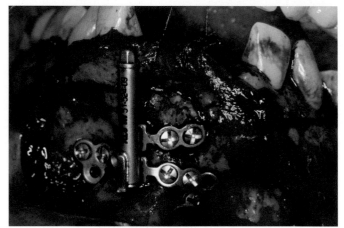

Fig. 7.15. The distractor is securely in place.

plate (Fig. 7.12). Also, the orientation of the saw should always be kept slightly angled toward the alveolar crest; this will prevent invasion of anatomical structures (i.e., the nasal spine, the nasal cavity, or the genial tubercules).

The bony segment is gently detached from the maxilla or mandible using a very fine chisel and mallet while holding the segment palatally or ligually with the finger (Fig. 7.13). At this point, the mobile segment is connected to the palatal or lingual gingiva only through the palatal/lingual periosteum. Once the segment is freed from the surrounding bone, the distractor is put back in place and secured through the use of screws that will engage in the predrilled holes previously mentioned (Fig. 7.14). A minimum number of five screws is recommended to secure the distractor (two screws for the upper segment and three screws for the lower segment).

These screws are self-drilling, but it is better to use the drill and predrill; this way, you will avoid running the risk of splitting the bony segment to be distracted. It is customary to use the 5-mm-length screws (Fig. 7.15).

Once the distractor is securely in place, it is useful to activate it and see how the bony segment glides upward (Fig. 7.16). This is critical because if there is an impediment to the smooth trajectory of the segment to be distracted, it should be corrected at this point. This is usually the case when the mesial and distal cuts are somewhat parallel to each other instead of being divergent. This can be corrected using a fine fissure bur. The distractor is put back in its inactive mode, and a small opening is made in the gingiva ("button hole") to allow for the passage of the distractor's arm (Fig. 7.17). The suturing is done in two layers, using chromic gut sutures (Figs. 7.18 and 7.19). The removable temporary partial denture is adjusted to fit the new clinical situation (Figs. 7.20 and 7.21).

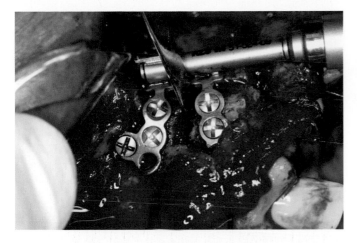

Fig. 7.16. The distractor is activated to make sure that there will be no interferences during the distraction process.

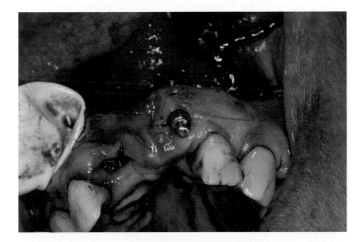

Fig. 7.17. After bringing back the segment to its original position, a small incision is made close to the gingival crest to accommodate the head of the distractor post.

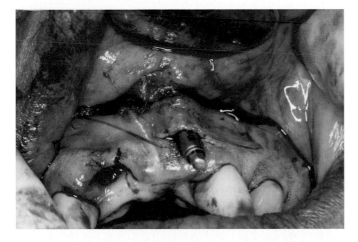

Fig. 7.18. A two-layer suturing technique is used to close the wound. First, the deeper layers (muscles, etc.) are sutured with an internal horizontal or vertical mattress suture. You must use resorbable material such as chromic gut for this first suture.

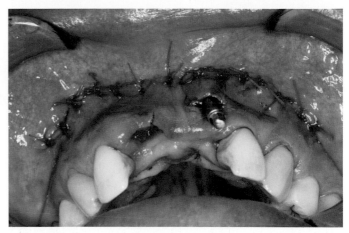

Fig. 7.19. Now that the deeper layers are sutured, the second layer will approximate the edges of the wound without tension and the area will heal by primary intention. You can use resorbable or nonresorbable material for this suture (here, 4-0 chromic gut was used).

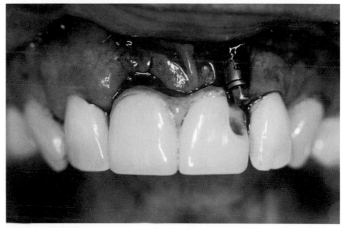

Fig. 7.20. The temporary removable prosthesis is adjusted, so that it will not interfere with the distractor. It will be grinded down gradually as the distraction progresses and the bone and tissues extend vertically.

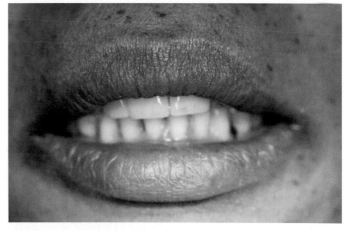

Fig. 7.21. The patient with the adjusted prosthesis in place. The device is not noticeable.

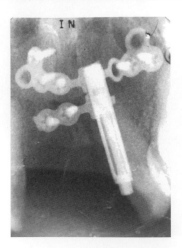

Fig. 7.22. Periapical radiograph of the segment at the end of the alveolar distraction process.

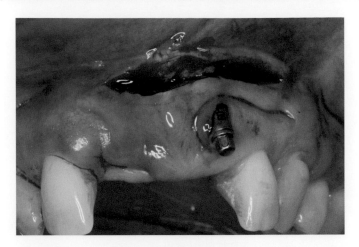

Fig. 7.24. Two months after the end of the distraction period, the device is removed using a smaller incision.

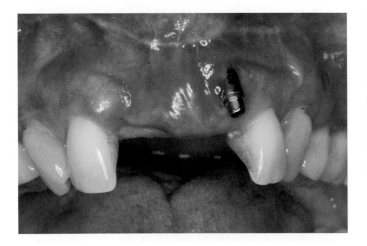

Fig. 7.23. The bone has been distracted to the desired length. We ask the patient to stop activating the device. In 2 months, the distractor will be removed.

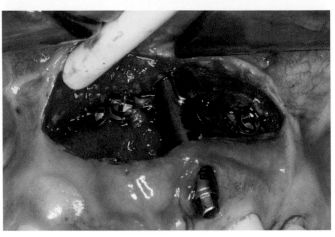

Fig. 7.25. The distractor is exposed by blunt dissection with a periosteal elevator.

The patient is seen 7 days after the surgery (latency period), and the distractor is then activated with one complete turn of the screw (0.3 mm) (starting of the distraction period). The patient is given the "distractor key" and asked to repeat the procedure twice a day (0.6 mm/day of distraction). The patient is monitored weekly until the desired vertical bone height is achieved (Figs. 7.22 and 7.23). At this point, the consolidation period begins.

This is a 3-month rest period that allows for bone remodeling and consolidation. After 2 months, the distractor is removed (Figs. 7.24 through 7.26), the wound is sutured, and the patient is sent home for another month (Fig. 7.27). At the end of the 3 months (2 + 1) of consolidation, the patient is sent for

a CT scan evaluation and the implants are placed. It is important to place the implants shortly after the removal of the distractor; otherwise, you may run the risk of losing the newly formed bone.

Technique for the Posterior Segment

The posterior segment is much more challenging (Fig. 7.28) than the anterior segments because of anatomical limitations, access, and proximity of vital structures (mandibular nerve, maxillary sinus). It is very useful to visualize the anatomy of the mandible using a plastic model (Fig. 7.29). This model (ClearView Anatomical Models; Medical Modeling LLC, Golden, CO) can be obtained after the CT scan is sent to the company (Fig. 7.30). The incisions are planned on this ex-

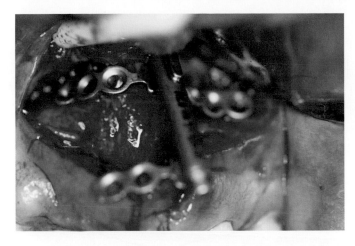

Fig. 7.26. The screws are removed, as well as the device. Notice the amount of bone gained in the vertical dimension in less than 1 month.

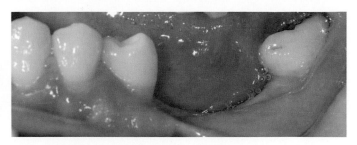

Fig. 7.28. A 30-year-old patient presenting with a posterior vertical height defect. Tooth No. 17 cannot be used as an abutment for a fixed or removable partial denture.

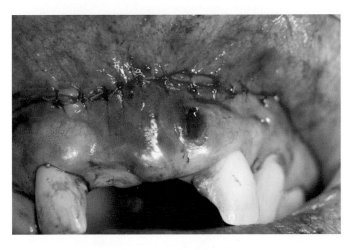

Fig. 7.27. The surgical wound is closed with internal and external sutures, as before, and the area is left to heal undisturbed for 1 month before placing the implants.

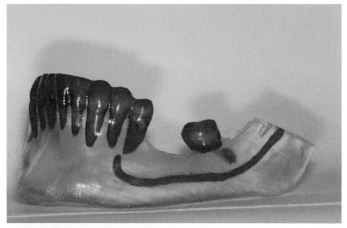

Fig. 7.29. An exact replica of the patient's mandible. This model (ClearView Anatomical Model; Medical Modeling LLC, Golden, CO, USA) obtained from the patient's CT scan will allow the critical landmarks (mental foramen, mandibular canal, roots, etc.) to be located precisely. This in turn will make for guess-free and stress-free surgery.

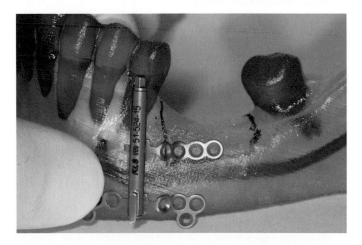

Fig. 7.30. Radiographic images (CT scan of the patient's mandible) showing the mandibular nerve, mental foramen, etc. Notice the posterior vertical bony ledge due to the alveolar bone loss and its distance from the mandibular nerve.

Alveolar Distraction Osteogenesis **123**

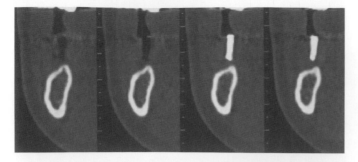

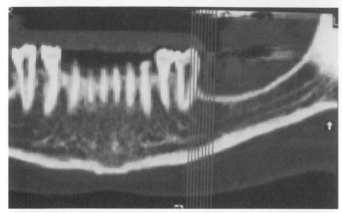

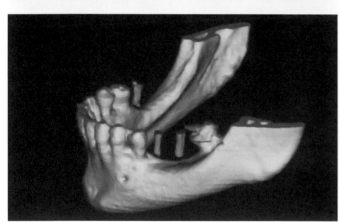

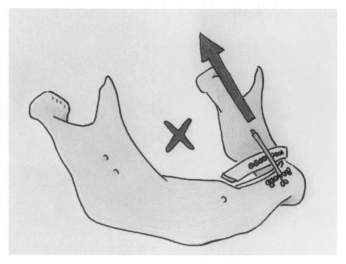

Fig. 7.32. The *arrow* shows an incorrect vector of distraction. The bony segment will be too lingual and therefore could not be used for proper dental implant placement.

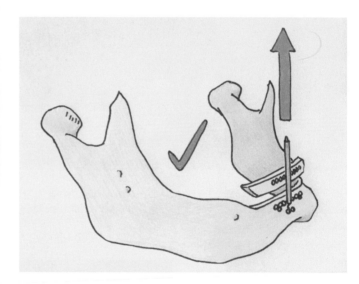

Fig. 7.31. The segment to be distracted is drawn on the model and will be replicated in the mouth precisely during the surgery. The distractor arms are modified and bent prior to the surgery to fit the clinical situation. This will save a lot of time and aggravation during the surgery.

Fig. 7.33. The *arrow* shows a correct vector of distraction. The bony segment will be distracted parallel with the long axis of the adjacent teeth. Dental implants can be placed in the proper alignment.

tremely accurate model, and the distractor is bent and adapted beforehand (Fig. 7.31). This will save considerable time, stress, and aggravation during the surgery.

A Few Words of Caution

- Pay special attention to the direction of the vector in the lower anterior mandibular region (Figs. 7.32 and 7.33).

- Make sure that the distractor does not interfere with the occlusion.

- Select patients who are reliable and compliant.

- Always "overdistract" by a couple of milimeters to ensure you will have enough bone.

Preoperative Instructions

- Antibiotherapy (i.e., amoxicillin 500 mg 3 times a day starting the day of surgery and for 7 days) is indicated.

- Mild oral sedation could be useful (i.e., diazepam 5 mg the night before and 5 mg 1 hour before the procedure).

- Analgesics are recommended (i.e., ibuprofen 600 mg 1 hour before the surgery).

Postoperative Instructions

- Corticosteroids for 5 days: dexamethasone 0.75 mg, 5 tablets the day of surgery, then 4 tablets the next day, then 3 tablets, and so on, to control the swelling

- Analgesics: acetaminophen with codeine (Tylenol #3) or ibuprofen 600 mg (Motrin 600) to control the pain

- Ice pack 20 minutes on/20 minutes off for the first 24 hours

- Chlorhexidine rinses twice a day for 7 days

Possible Complications

- Possible necrosis of the bony segment if it is too small or completely detached from the periosteum

- Fibrous tissue formation at the end of the traction period: this is more likely to occur if the traction has been too vigorous (i.e., 1 mm/day or more)

- Infection

- Fracture of transport segment

- Fracture of anchorage segment

- Premature consolidation

- Undesirable transport vector

- Fracture of the distraction rod or of the transport disc (Mazzonetto and Torrezan, 2003)

REFERENCES

Birch, J.G., and M.L. Samchukov. 2004. Use of the Ilizarov method to correct lower limb deformities in children and adolescents. *J. Am. Acad. Orthop. Surg.* 12(3):144–154.

Block, M.S., A. Chang, and C. Crawford. 1996. Mandibular alveolar ridge augmentation in the dog using distraction osteogenesis. *J. Oral Maxillofac. Surg.* 54(3):309–314.

Chiapasco, M., U. Consolo, A. Bianchi, and P. Ronchi. 2004. Alveolar distraction osteogenesis for the correction of vertically deficient edentulous ridges: a multicenter prospective study on humans. *Int. J. Oral Maxillofac. Implants* 19(3):399–407.

Chin, M., and B.A. Toth. 1996. Distraction osteogenesis in maxillofacial surgery using internal devices: review of five cases. *J. Oral Maxillofac. Surg.* 54(1):45–53.

Cope, J.B., and M.L. Samchukov. 2001. Mineralization dynamics of regenerate bone during mandibular osteodistraction. *Int. J. Oral Maxillofac. Surg.* 30(3):234–242.

Dibart, S., and M. Karima. 2006. *Practical Periodontal Plastic Surgery.* Blackwell Publishing, Ames, IA.

Ilizarov, G.A. 1971. Basic principles of transosseous compression and distraction osteosynthesis. *Orthop. Travmatol. Protez.* 32(11):7–15.

Mazzonetto, R., M. Allais, P.E. Maurette, and R.W. Moreira. 2007. A retrospective study of the potential complications during alveolar distraction osteogenesis in 55 patients. *J. Oral Maxillofac. Surg.* 36:6–10.

McCarthy, J.G., D.A. Staffenberg, R.J. Wood, C.B. Cutting, B.H. Gray, and T.H. Thorne. 1995. Introduction of an intra-oral bone lengthening device. *Plast. Reconstr. Surg.* 96(4):978–981.

Ortiz Monasterio, F., F. Molina, L. Andrade, O. Rodriguez, and J. Sainz Arregui. 1997. Simultaneous mandibular and maxillary distraction in hemifacial microsomia in adults: avoiding occlusal disasters. *Plast. Reconstr. Surg.* 100(4):852–861.

Samchukov, M.L., J.B. Cope, R.B. Harper, and J.D. Ross. 1998. Biomechanical considerations of mandibular lengthening and widening by gradual distraction using a computer model. *J. Oral Maxillofac. Surg.* 56(1):51–59.

Chapter 8 Papillary Construction After Dental Implant Therapy

Peyman Shahidi, DDS, MScD, Serge Dibart, DMD,

and Yun Po Zhang, PhD, DDS(hon)

HISTORY

The presence of a "black triangle" due to the absence of inter-proximal papilla between two adjacent implants has become a steady concern among implant surgeons and restorative dentists. Three main surgical methods have been proposed in the past at second-stage surgery (uncovering) to correct the problem. Palacci in 1995 suggested that a full-thickness flap be raised from the palatal side of the implant and a portion of it be rotated 90 degrees to accommodate the interproximal space of the implant. Possible compromise of the blood supply of the rotated small flap, limited amount of pedunculated soft tissue for some larger interproximal areas, and lack of keratinized tissue in cases with a narrow band of attached gingiva on the facial seem to be some of the limitations of this technique. In 1999, Adriaenssens et al. introduced a novel flap design, the "palatal sliding strip flap," to help form papillae between implants and between natural teeth on the anterior area of the maxilla. The flap was designed and managed in a way that allowed the palatal mucosa to slide in a labial direction after dissection of two mesial and distal strips (to create papillae and at the same time augment the labial ridge).

Nemcovsky et al. in 2000 introduced a U-shaped flap raised toward the buccal; the nature of this design was essentially the same as the one introduced earlier by Adriaenssens, with some minor differences. In 2004, Misch et al. modified Nemcovsky et al.'s technique further by raising the U-shaped flap toward the palatal rather than the buccal side. In 2004, Shahidi developed a surgical procedure with the goal of guiding the soft tissue that formerly covered the implant over to the sides of the implant and to gently squeeze this piece of tissue after insertion of the healing abutment. This was done to provide enough soft tissue in the interproximal spaces to allow for papilla generation.

In brief, there is not one single technique that is universally accepted to be the one that works 100% of the time. Tissue engineering, with the implantation of fibroblasts in the papillary area, may, in the future, help solve this problem by providing more predictability.

INDICATIONS

- At second-stage dental implant uncovering, between an implant and a tooth or between two or more implants, to minimize the formation of a "black triangle"

- Thick periodontal biotype

CONTRAINDICATIONS

- Thin periodontal biotype

- Lack of keratinized gingiva around the implant(s)

- Need to correct underlying bone

ARMAMENTARIUM

- A basic surgical set as described in *Practical Periodontal Plastic Surgery*

- Implant kit

- Healing abutments

TECHNIQUE

In the single implant model, a small U-shaped flap is created to allow mobilization of the tissue in the mesial direction. Another U-shaped flap, mirror image of the first one and sharing the same buccolingual incision, allows mobilization of the tissues to the distal direction. Occlusally, these full- or partial-thickness U-shaped flaps form an H-shape design (Fig. 8.1). The exact

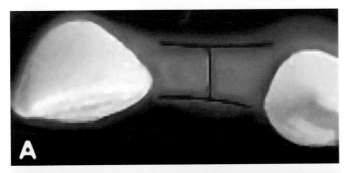

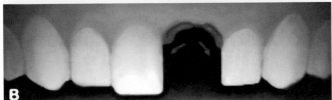

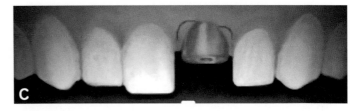

Fig. 8.1. Diagram showing the uncovering incision and procedures for a single implant occlusally (**a**) and buccally (**b**) and with the healing abutment in place (**c**).

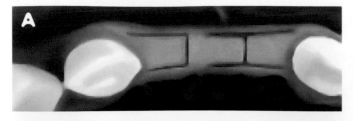

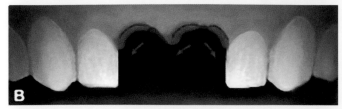

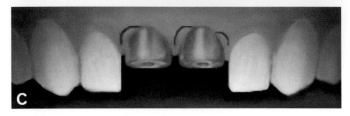

Fig. 8.2. Diagram showing the uncovering incision and procedures for two implants side by side, occlusally (**a**) and bucally (**b**) with the healing abutments in place (**c**).

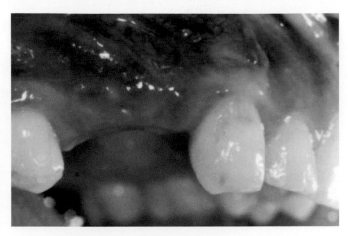

Fig. 8.3. Before uncovering of implant Nos. 4 and 5.

location of the implant is obtained using periapical/bitewing radiographs in combination with alveolar ridge mapping with an explorer following local anesthesia.

In a multiple implant model (Fig. 8.2), the covering tissue of the most mesial implant provides the proximal papilla (i.e., mesial) of that implant using the U-shape design; the second implant provides the contralateral papilla (i.e., distal) of the first implant.

After proper local anesthesia (Fig. 8.3), the initial incisions, made using a No. 15 blade, are done as follows:

1. The first incision is done in a buccopalatal–lingual direction. The location ranges from the distal edge of the platform of the implant to the middle of the platform, depending upon the amount of tissue needed between implants or between implant and adjacent tooth.

2. The second step involves the placement of a mesiodistal incision on the buccal side for each implant, perpendicular to the first buccolingual incision. The incision is continued in a slight parabola buccally when there is adequate keratinized gingiva on the buccal to create a gingival margin around the implant. The incision is continued in a slight parabola palatally if there is insufficient keratinized gingiva on the buccal. Precautions must be taken to preserve buccal keratinized tissue. The incision passes the mesial

or distal platform of the implant and ends halfway between the platform and the adjacent implant or tooth.

3. The third step involves the placement of a mesiodistal incision on the lingual/palatal parallel to the incision on the buccal. The incision for the anterior implants curves slightly off buccally in the middle, as the top of the papilla should be smaller than its base in the buccolingual direction. In posterior implants, the incision is also placed slightly palatally because the width of the platform of a posterior implant is usually smaller than the width of its crown. This is essential in gaining an adequate buccolingual/palatal papilla or col width to cover the interproximal space.

4. Flaps are elevated by using the tip of the blade and the tip of an Orban knife. First, the soft tissues are reflected from the underlying implant; then each mini-flap is undermined by the No. 15 blade and the Orban knife, and the full- or partial-thickness mini-flap is extended to about 1 mm from the adjacent implant or tooth.

Flaps are mobilized and pushed in the mesial and distal directions to open a "window" and place the healing abutment. The application of gauze in the area for a few minutes facilitates the molding of the tissues while pushing the tissues to the sides. After removing the cover screw, a healing abutment with proper height, width, and shape is inserted into the implant with or without a provisional restoration. This shapes the future papilla by pushing the tissues to the sides and holding them upright (Figs. 8.4 and 8.5). The same technique is repeated for implant(s) distal to the first implant. No sutures are applied, because healing abutments hold the tissues in the proper position.

The patient then receives postoperative instructions and is scheduled for a follow-up visit within 7 to 10 days.

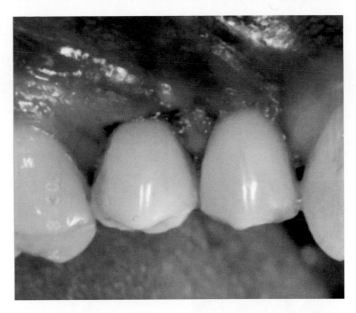

Fig. 8.4. The abutment and provisional restorations for Nos. 4 and 5 in place. Notice how the gingiva has been folded and maintained via the temporary restorations.

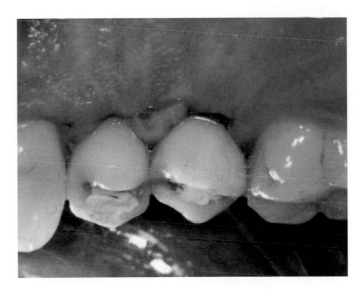

Fig. 8.5. The palatal view. The U- and H-shaped flaps have been folded, creating papillae.

POSTOPERATIVE INSTRUCTIONS

The patient is advised to rinse with chlorhexidine gluconate (PerioGard oral rinse; Colgate Palmolive) twice daily for 1 week and take ibuprofen (Advil) 200 mg in case of discomfort. Postsurgical care after the first week of healing involves regular brushing with a soft bristle toothbrush (Colgate 360-degree toothbrush) and rinsing for another week with chlorhexidine gluconate.

SURGICAL INDEXING

This should be considered to increase predictability and aesthetic outcome.

POSSIBLE COMPLICATIONS

- Complications are very unusual due to the minimally invasive nature of the procedure.

- Infection is always a possibility and should be treated with local antibiotherapy and antiseptic mouth rinses.

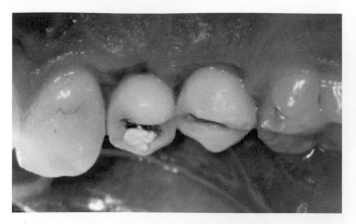

Fig. 8.6. Two weeks postoperatively. The area has healed uneventfully.

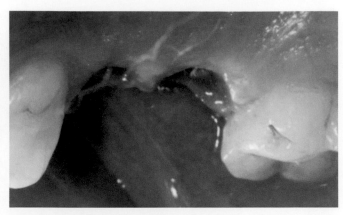

Fig. 8.8. Five months postoperatively (palatal view). Notice the presence of a papilla between implant Nos. 4 and 5.

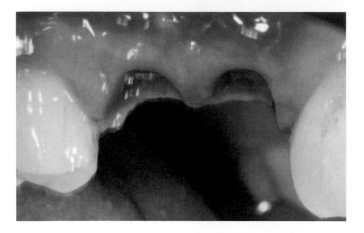

Fig. 8.7. Five months postoperatively. Notice the formation of the papilla between implant Nos. 4 and 5.

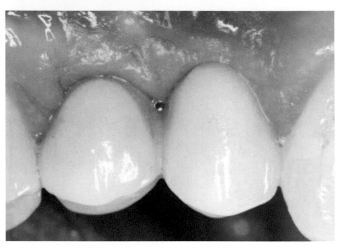

Fig. 8.9. Area with the final restorations at 20 months postoperatively.

HEALING

The results are very stable 1.5 years postsurgery (Figs. 8.6 through 8.9).

The efficacy of this new uncovering technique compared with the conventional one for papilla generation has been tested on 33 patients with 67 implants that were adjacent to either teeth or implants (Shahidi 2004). The mean difference between the two surgical methods revealed that this new technique provided 1.5 mm greater papilla height ($P < .001$) than the conventional one (mean difference for height of a papilla between an implant and a tooth was 1.71 mm [$P < .001$], mean difference papilla height between implants was 0.78 mm [$P < .138$] at 6 months). The papilla generation between an implant and a tooth was more stable and predictable than papilla generation between two implants.

REFERENCES

Adriaenssens, P., M. Hermans, A. Ingber, V. Prestipino, P. Daelemans, and C. Malevez. 1999. Palatal sliding strip flap: soft tissue management to restore maxillary anterior esthetics at stage 2 surgery: a clinical report. *Int. J. Oral Maxillofac. Implants* 14:30–36.

Dibart, S., and M. Karima. 2006. *Practical Periodontal Plastic Surgery.* Blackwell Publishing, Ames, IA.

Misch, C.E., K.E. Al Shammori, and H.L. Wang. 2004. Creation of inter-implant papillae through split finger technique. *Implant Dent.* 13:20–27.

Nemcovsky, C.E., O. Moses, and Z. Artzi. 2000. Interproximal papillae reconstruction in maxillary implants. *J. Periodontol.* 71:308–314.

Palacci, P. 1995. *Optimal Implant Positioning and Soft Tissue Management for the Branemark System.* Quintessence, Chicago, pp. 35–39.

Shahidi, P. Efficacy of a new papilla generation technique in implantology. MS thesis. Boston University. Boston 2004.

Chapter 9 Dental Implant Placement Including the Use of Short Implants

Albert Price, DMD, MS, and Ming Fang Su, DMD, MS

HISTORY

Branemark's exploration of the vascular supply to healing bone evolved into the concept referred to as *osseointegration*. The physical design of his prototype dental implant was made of titanium that was milled into a cylindrical screw form with a tapered apical end and a coronal flared neck topped by a circular platform. A hex nut was milled into the corona and a screw chamber was bored and tapped through this into the body of the implant for fixation of external devices (Fig. 9.1).

A full-thickness flap was reflected and the bone crest exposed. The implant was placed by preparing a cylindrical hole through the compact bone of the crest and extending it to engage cortex at the base of the mandible, floor of the nose, or the floor of the sinus.

The osteotomy represented the body of the implant without threads (Figs. 9.2 and 9.3) Threads were tapped into the sides of the osteotomy when necessary, and the entry was countersunk to match the screw threads and the flared neck of the implant. A cover screw was placed over the external hex platform to seal the attachment chamber. The entire preparation was done with careful attention to measurement so that the finished installation lay flush with the bone surface. The entry flap was then sutured passively with the partial dissection marginal incision providing primary connective tissue approximation and rapid healing.

Branemark's surgical technique required adherence to certain principles based on his teams studies:

1. Atraumatic bone preparation with attention to minimizing heat production: constant irrigation

2. Primary surgical stability achieved with bicortical stabilization where possible (upper anterior/lower anterior)

3. Spacing of multiple implants: 7.0 to 7.5 mm on center

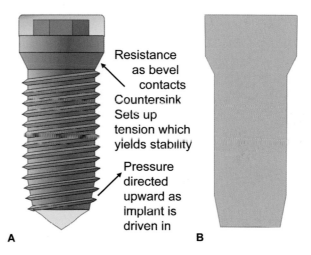

Fig. 9.2 A, Osteotomy outline followed by implant placement (cylindrical shape). **B,** Outline of implant that will fit the osteotomy site.

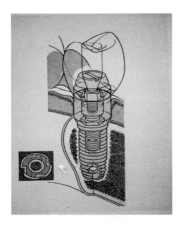

Fig. 9.1 Image of a Branemark implant depicting design and surface structure. (Reprinted with permission from Branemark PI, et al. 1985. *Tissue-Integrated Prostheses.* Quintessence, Chicago.)

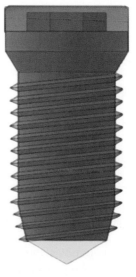

Fig. 9.3 Implant fitted into the osteotomy site (cylindrical shape).

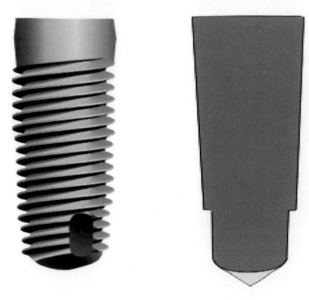

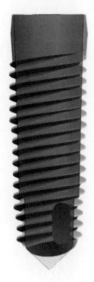

Fig. 9.5 Tapered implant within the osteotomy site.

Fig. 9.4 Tapered implant and outline of osteotomy site.

4. Provide healing interval with no direct load to allow undisturbed osseointegration

Most of these early implants were placed in the mandibule between the mental foramina and maxillary anterior/bicuspid regions. The objective was to offer an alternative to an inadequate removable prosthesis.

Implants have become a standard of care and the treatment of choice for replacement of missing teeth. All areas of the mouth have been restored, and while the threaded implant is still the dominant form, the cylindrical shape and the attachment platform have evolved.

Three basic forms that are available are the cylinder with screw threads (Branemark's design), the tapered cylinder with threads (e.g., Zimmer [Figs. 9.4 and 9.5]), and the tapered form without threads, which is press fit (Bicon [Fig. 9.6] and Endopore). The internal architecture of the bone influences the effectiveness of these forms to gain the necessary stability at time of placement.

Branemark stressed bicortical stabilization as a method to secure his implant system. His mechanical shape creates stability by the resistance of the countersink to the draw or pull of the threads into the bony preparation (Fig. 9.2A); this requires heavy compact bone at each end of the osteotomy. To ensure maximum use of bone and bicortical engagement (CT was not available then), the suggestion was made to place the finger firmly against the base of the mandible and to feel that the bur had penetrated the cortex. In the maxillary anterior, one was to place the finger in the nasal areas to feel the penetration of the floor of the nose (cortex). If the internal

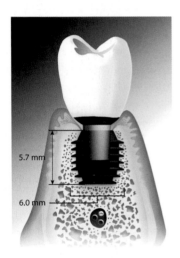

Fig. 9.6 Bicon short implant (5.7 × 6 mm) placed in the mandible (especially useful in cases with insufficient bony height).

architecture had trabeculae of sufficient bulk, then the engagement of the more compact border areas was not needed. However, if the trabeculae were thin and widely spaced, such as in the upper and lower posterior, then the screw pressures could break or strip the bone threads in the body and apex area of the implant or collapse the coronal bevel and result in a "spinner." It is possible to engage the cortex at the floor of the sinus and the top of the mandibular canal, but this is often not desirable.

As the scope of placement widened to include the posterior areas and single tooth sites, the need for alternate mechanics of surgical stability evolved.

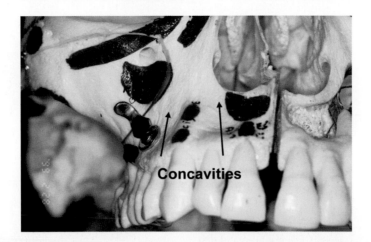

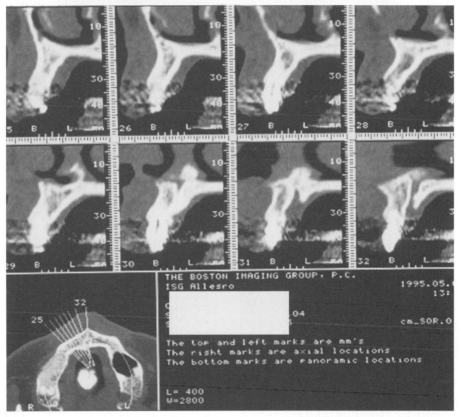

Fig. 9.7 Dry scull and CT scan showing specific anatomic features and trabeculation of the maxillary bone.

Originally designed to fit tapered cross sectional sites (areas with depressions like the incisal fossa and the depression over the upper first bicuspid) the tapered form is especially useful in areas of light, thin trabeculation (Fig. 9.7)

The tapered screw form provides an alternative method of achieving surgical stability. Its wedge-shaped screw form achieves compression of the tapered osteotomy along its entire surface (see Figs. 9.4 and 9.5).

INDICATIONS

Dental implants are used to:

1. Replace individual teeth

2. Support fixed and removable prostheses

3. Anchor maxillofacial prosthesis

4. Act as anchorage for orthodontic movement

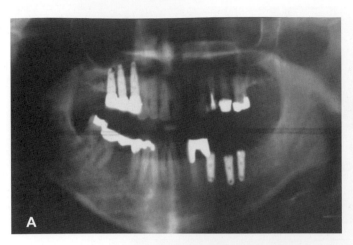

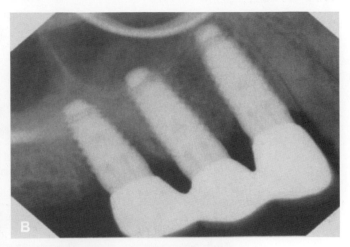

Fig. 9.8 **A,** Panoramic radiograph (distortion ±25%). **B,** Periapical radiograph (distortion ±15%).

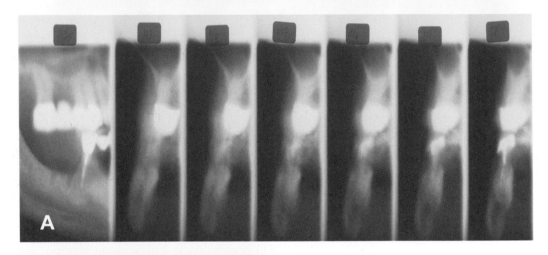

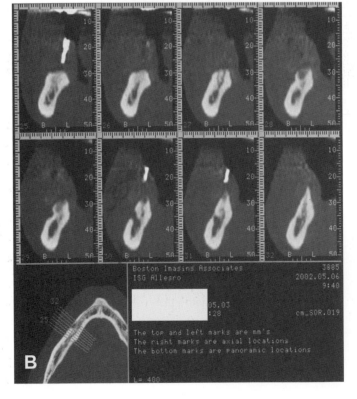

TECHNIQUE

Anesthesia

Block anesthesia is the most efficient. Marcaine supplemented with lidocaine provides 3 to 4 hours of good working anesthesia with minimal local reinforcement. Some practitioners prefer only infiltration so that the patient "feels" the proximity to vital structures and thus avoid potential damage to nerves. With a distortion level of 1% or less, the reformatted CT images, coupled with a surgeon's "feel" for anatomy, can be used with confidence (Figs. 9.8 and 9.9).

IMPLANT PLACEMENT

Entry Incision

The objective is to expose the bone where the osteotomy is to be placed and to minimize vascular disruption to sensitive bone areas (Fig. 9.10).

Fig. 9.9 **A,** Tomograph: "foggy" quality and slice thickness distort image. **B,** CT scan: distortion ±1%.

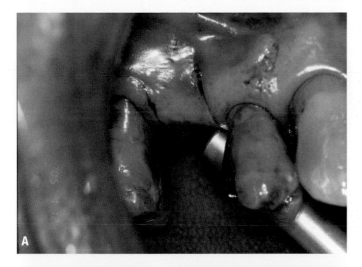

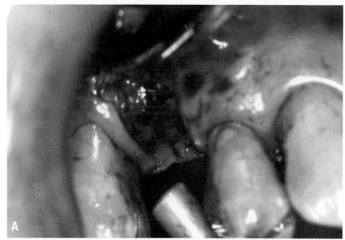

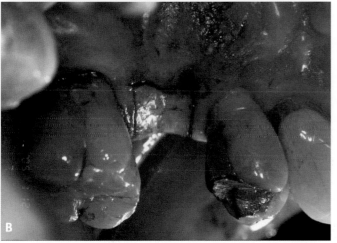

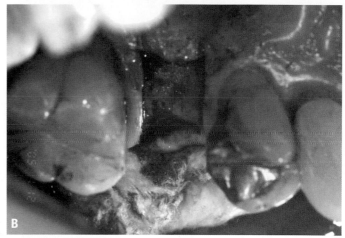

Fig. 9.10 Incision design buccally (**A**) and palatally (**B**) before the placement of implant No. 4.

Fig. 9.11 Full-thickness flap is reflected, exposing the alveolar crest, (**A**), buccally and (**B**), palatally.

Incisions vary with site objective and history of local trauma.

1. If one-stage implant or immediate load, a mid crestal incision with intrasulcular extensions buccally and lingually is used.

2. If classic delayed, two-stage implant, then

   - In the maxillary arch, a horizontal incision is usually made just to the palatal of line angles and two vertical incisions sparing the proximal papillae are extended through the mucogingival junction (MGJ) on the buccal. The flap is reflected into the vestibule and no retraction is needed (Fig. 9.11).

   - In the mandibular arch, an incision is made just to the buccal of line angles, or if the MGJ is close to this area, the incision is made below the MGJ and reverse split for about 2 mm to leave a small bed of periosteum behind. Vertical incisions sparing the papillae are extended over the crest and through the lingual MGJ. The flap is re-

flected to the lingual and usually buckles over onto itself, avoiding need for retraction.

3. If dealing with multiple implants in a severely resorbed lower arch with no vestibular depth, then an incision is made in middle of available keratinized tissue, reflecting enough to expose the crest.

SITE PREPARATION

The only time one needs to reduce bone at the site is a requirement for increased interocclusal space. It should be kept in mind that reducing the bone increases the crown-root ratio of the prosthesis, which increases stress-strain relationships at the abutment–implant interface.

The Osteotomy: Single Implant

The central goal is to have the implant perpendicular to the plane of occlusion, in the center of the occlusal table of the respective tooth form, and to have at least 1 mm of bone on

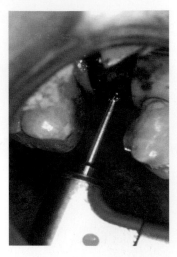

Fig. 9.12 Using a round bur, future site of implant osteotomy is marked.

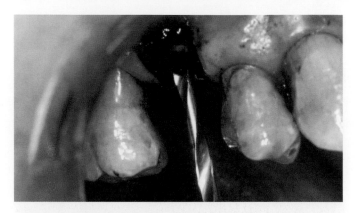

Fig. 9.13 Pilot drill is used to initiate the osteotomy.

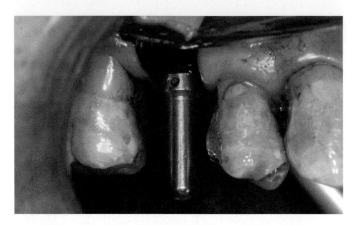

Fig. 9.14 Directional guide shows the proper alignment of the implant buccally.

all sides of implant. It is estimated that at least 0.5 mm of bone is necrosed in the most careful surgery (Rhinelander 1974a, 1974b).

Preparation

1. Using a small round bur (Fig. 9.12), the mesial–distal, buccal–lingual location is marked with a small depression. This is remeasured and accepted or changed, and then the crest is deepened for 2 to 3 mm with copious irrigation to penetrate the crestal cortex. In some sites, after penetrating 1 to 2 mm, the bur may suddenly drop (upper and lower posterior). If this happens, a perioprobe should be inserted and pushed until resistance is detected. The probe may drop 10 mm in areas of very little trabecular content. Caution during preparation should be used to achieve surgical stability.

2. The starting cylinder bur is usually 2.0 to 2.5 mm in diameter (Fig. 9.13), but in very dense bone, the addition of a 1.5-mm bur is useful. The burs should have guide marks to mark vertical depth, and these should be checked against a common rule (periodontal probe) for actual depth and reference to CT scan measurements. Many drill systems do not count the bevel at tip of bur, and the markings may not represent millimeters but instead a preferred depth for ideal placement of the implant. (It is assumed that a CT scan or some method of judging distance to vital structure has been used in treatment planning.)

At this stage, it is prudent to drill only as deep as needed to check vertical angulation (7 to 8 mm) with a direction guide. If a change is to be made, then it should be done before proceeding to larger drills. Sometimes it is necessary to use the round bur again to force this change. The direction guide with string attached is then placed (Figs. 9.14 and 9.15). The cylinder bur is aligned with this guide and then changed to

the new direction. The guide is pulled and the correction is made. Once the new direction is acceptable, the site is drilled to final depth. If vertical bone allows, overdrill the depth of the site by about 1.0 mm in the initial drill steps. This allows more flexibility as larger burs are used because they are not efficient end-cutters and can generate heat if pushed too hard trying to achieve increased depth at later stages. (Internally irrigated burs have not been found practical because they constantly clog and irrigation fails.)

Once the initial burs have created place and angulation, the site is gradually enlarged to the final size according to the steps recommended by the implant system guide.

WARNING: DRILL SPEED: Each drill system has been engineered to be run at certain speeds; failure to follow recommendations may overheat bone. Irrigation should be constant and drilling is done in a pumping action to remove bone filings, especially in very compact bone. (In the lower anterior, it is sometimes necessary to change to a new bur after one osteotomy; remember that the smaller burs are being used in every case.)

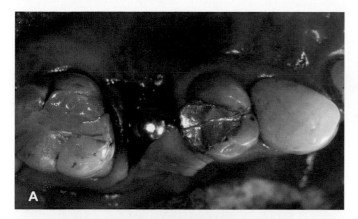

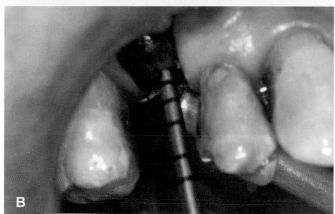

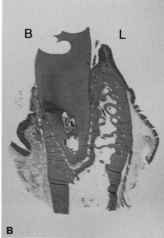

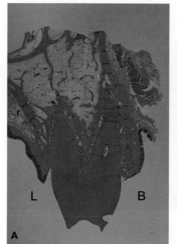

Fig. 9.16 Internal architecture. **A,** Maxillary bicuspid. **B,** Mandibular first bicuspid. Note different cortex and trabecular thickness. B, buccal area; L, lingual area.

Fig. 9.15 A, Directional guide shows the proper alignment of the implant occlusally. **B,** Using a periodontal probe, the proper depth of the osteotomy is being assessed.

During the final drill stages, a judgment needs to be made about whether to tap threads. Reflecting on the internal arrangement of trabeculae seen in the pictures (Figs. 9.16 and 9.17), it is possible to start "soft" and end "hard" as the last bur encounters heavy trabeculation or the inner aspect of bordering cortex or the residual compact socket from a recently extracted tooth.

If tapping threads is necessary, it should be done by hand or very low handpiece speed; the same speed used for placement of the implant (30 to 50 rpm). After tapping threads, the osteotomy should be flushed free of debris and then restimulated to bleed by probing the apical area.

In some systems, a final shaping is needed to countersink or prepare for a slightly enlarged collar. If resistance or drill debris has been minimal during the preparation, then one can eliminate or reduce these last steps. If implant site is not bleeding enough to fill the site after any of these steps, then have the patient open and close several times after stimulating with a probe. This "pumps" the maxillary artery and results in the desired fill with natural fluids.

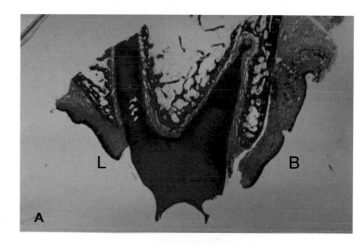

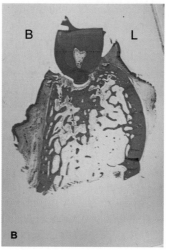

Fig. 9.17 Internal architecture of furcation area of first molars. **A,** Maxillary first molar. **B,** Mandibular first molar. Note differences in cortex and trabecular dimensions at the maxillary versus mandibular sites. B, buccal area; L, lingual area.

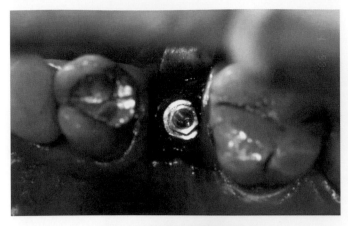

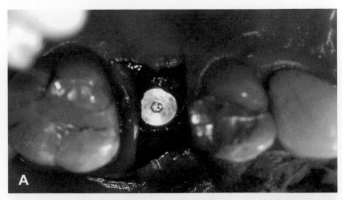

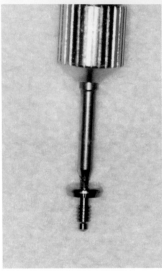

Fig. 9.18 The cover screw is used to seal the coronal portion of the implant before flap closure.

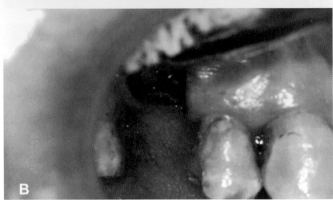

Fig. 9.19 A, Cover screw is seated. B, Implant is at level or below alveolar crest.

FIXTURE INSTALLATION

The implant fixture may be placed by hand or with a controlled drill speed and torque. A torque-metered speed of 30 to 50 rpm is preferred with torque set at a low value to start. The drilling sequence used to prepare the site should give one a sense of the torque needed. If one is in doubt, it is best to start with low torque of 15 to 20 N/cm. If the insertion stalls, then reverse drill for a half turn and proceed with next highest torque. This clears the treads. Note should be made of final insertion torque on record, and this is used to determine waiting period for integration and/or loading. Hand installation does not have this objective measure of torque, but sometimes it is preferred in very "delicate" sites. Hand insertion with an unmetered ratchet wrench is discouraged because excess stress can fracture buccal plates and/or strip threading or overcompress site. A surgical insertion torque of 20 N/cm would probably call for a 6-month wait while 35 to 45 N/cm could be loaded immediately. Experience will guide in this judgment. After the fixture is adjusted to its final position, either a cover screw or healing abutment is placed. If trabeculation is light or thin and insertion torque is minimal, then a passive healing is required and the final result should be at or slightly below crest with cover screw in place (Figs. 9.18 and 9.19).

POSSIBLE PROBLEMS AND COMPLICATIONS

Common Drilling Problems

1. *Underdrill of site depth:* This can result in thread stripping as implant bottoms before engaging bevel; pertains to Branemark style hex top with countersunk neck or rapid taper like the Astra ST

2. *Excess drill speed:* Burns bone, kills osteocytes, and results in early fixture loss

3. *Failure to "read" bone external contours:* Perforation of buccal or lingual (Figs. 9.7 and 9.20). This can be very dangerous with postoperative swelling and closure of airway in case of lingual lower cuspid site; roughly the area where the sublingual gland is located; see multiple vascular supplies to this area (Fig. 9.22)

4. *Tipping of drill* as depth increases from use of finger rest on tooth and rotating around rest instead of vertical pumping movement

5. *Overdrilling depth* or *irregular uneven osteotomy* can result in loss of implant into the sinus (Fig. 9.21) or within the mandible when there is a "hollow" anatomy

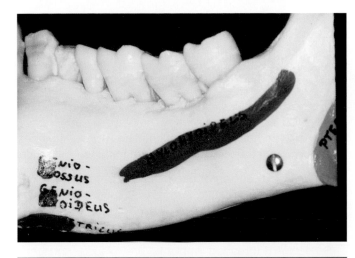

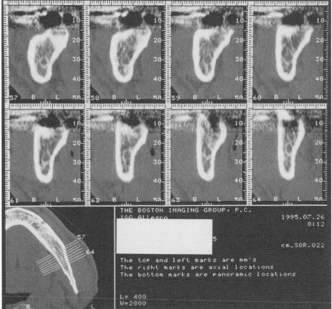

Fig. 9.20 Mylohyoid insertion line and canal proximity can limit angle of implant placement.

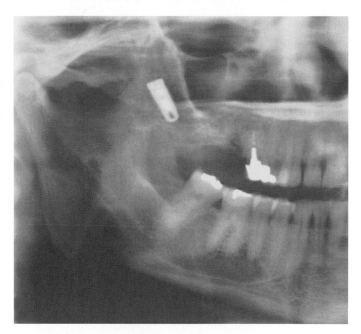

Fig. 9.21 Implant accidentally displaced into the maxillary sinus.

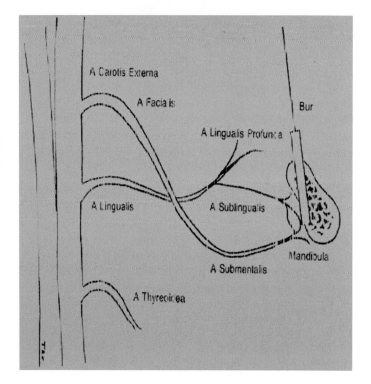

Fig. 9.22 Diagram showing sublingual and submental arteries that can be injured during implant placement in the canine/premolar area due to the presence of a lingual concavity. (Reprinted with permission from *JOMI* 1993;8[3]:329-333.)

In addition to drilling problems, several local site variables may complicate placement. These include:

1. Slopes mesial–distal and/or buccal–lingual or both

2. Vestibular depth may be very shallow (1 to 2 mm)

3. Thin cortex at crest and thin trabeculae internally (maxillary posterior)

4. Dense 1- to 2-mm crest and very poor internal trabecular distribution (mandibular posterior; especially after failed bridge where pontic has covered site)

5. Inadequate vertical height; maxillary first molar/sinus, lower posterior over canal

6. Buccal concavities: incisal fossa, cuspid fossa (Figs. 9.7 and 9.20)

7. Lingual concavities: submandibular, sublingual gland areas (Figs. 9.20 and 9.22)

Slopes: Major discrepancies in site platform (mesial–distal or buccal–lingual) should be corrected with grafting. Minor

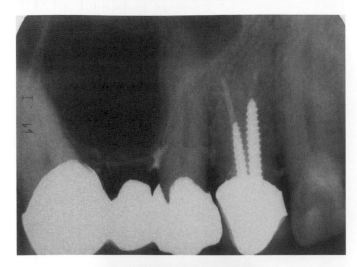

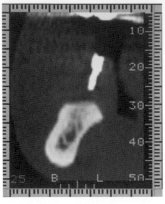

Fig. 9.23 Anatomic limits. Sinus extension, resulting in less than 1 mm bone at the alveolar crest (*top*). Crestal resorption: there is less than 7 mm bone above the mandibular canal, impairing standard implant placement (*bottom*).

bone level, the implants can be left above the floor and still retain maximum bone integration. It is even possible to leave the majority of the bevel above the crest, but this must be planned ahead and use of mid crestal incision is necessary.

Thin bone and minimal internal support: The site can be underdrilled (stop one drill short of final), laterally compressed with osteotomes, or site abandoned and allowed to reheal or even grafted internally and revisited at 3 to 4 months.

Inadequate vertical height: Site can be grafted with a block graft, or short implants with increased surface area can be used (Fig. 9.23).

Buccal concavities: This can present the most difficulty. Sometimes threaded implants are placed and then grafted. The implant may be placed at an acute angle and restored with an angled abutment. This often results in a "knee" at gingival margin, which then recedes and can expose the restorative margin. Another alternative in multiple site cases is to skip this site and bridge it with a pontic.

Lingual concavities: In the mandibular second molar, one can change the angle with the direction following the buccal plate. It is necessary to avoid encroachment on tongue space. Lower cuspid lingual concavity has multiple vascular supply, so it is very dangerous to perforate this area, with the potential for submylohyoid swelling and closure of airspace (see Fig. 9.22).

Multiple sites: Most of the issues with multiple sites are solved by good prosthetic guidance. In general, the implants need to be placed in the center of the crown shape to be supported in a buccal–lingual and mesial–distal manner.

The limits of placement proximity are different for implant-to-implant versus implant-to-tooth.

The general rule is to have at least 2 mm of bone between. This is problematic for two reasons: Tarnow et al. (2003) published data supporting the need for at least 3 mm to support interdental papillae. This would apply to Branemark-style implants where the cupping of adjacent implants would overlap and drop interproximal bone and the soft tissue above—the interproximal papillae. Other style implants may not present this problem. If one is dealing with heavy compact bone such as in the lower anterior, then placing implants too close endangers the endosseous vascular supply between them and there is the risk of bone necrosis between and loss of both implants and bone.

Implants can be placed closer to teeth because they have a greater vascular net in their PDL, which is connected through numerous holes to the adjacent marrow.

It may be more prudent to skip an implant and bridge a site if mesial–distal proximity becomes a problem. For ex-

contour differences can be adjusted for by interplay between implant anatomy and site anatomy. For example, if a site has a 2-mm deficiency from mid crest to buccal line angles, then a Branemark style implant can be used by placing the implant at the level of the lingual crest. This intentionally leaves the buccal bevel exposed, but at 1 year, this bone would have been lost in the cupping resorption usually seen with this style implant. As long as the palatal bone and half the mesial and distal bone serve the purpose of creating surgical stability, the implant placement can be left at a reasonable height and the C/R ratio is not affected.

Minimal vestibular depth: This often happens in the lower anterior with severe resorption, classic Branemark case. If the crest was leveled and the implants are placed by the standard protocol, then the connections could fall below the floor and vestibular depth. By ignoring the buccal and lingual slopes and seating implants at mesial and distal

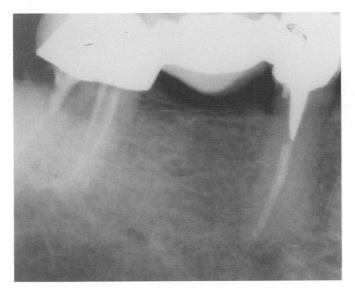

Fig. 9.24 Periapical radiograph showing mandibular molar necessitating extraction and replacement with implants. Due to insufficient vertical bony height above the mandibular canal, short implants were selected to restore missing dentition.

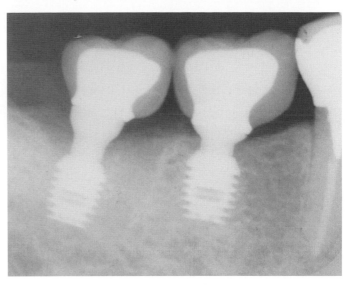

Fig. 9.26 Periapical radiograph showing implants restored.

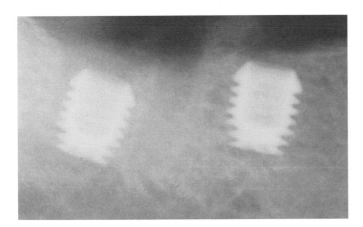

Fig. 9.25 Short implants (Bicon, Boston, MA, USA) were placed to overcome vertical limitation.

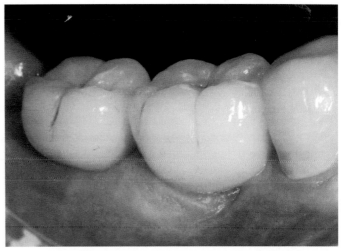

Fig. 9.27 Clinical picture of restored short implants.

ample, in the upper anterior, it might be better to skip the lateral site if inadequate spacing exists and/or to use the lateral and skip the central position if an overly large incisal foramen is present.

Short implants: In the past several years, the statistical analysis has shown decreased success rates with implants less than 10 mm. This is being challenged by newer forms and changed surface textures and treatments. Roughened surfaces, square threads, and plate form implants with greater surface area have been used successfully (Gentile 2005). While success rates may not be 100%, it is still possible and judicious to use short implants in select cases, especially when patients refuse extensive graft placement (Figs. 9.24 through 9.29).

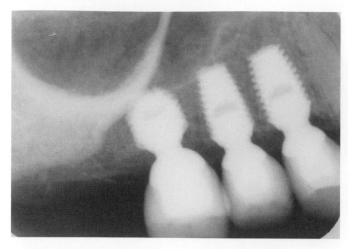

Fig. 9.28 Short implants were used to overcome the anatomical limitations of sinus proximity (avoiding extensive sinus grafting).

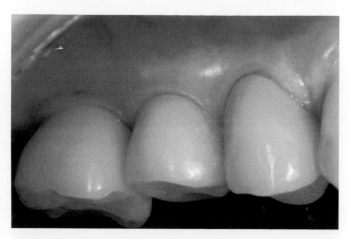

Fig. 9.29 Clinical picture of final implant-supported restoration.

REFERENCES

Gentile, M., S.K. Chuang, and T. Dodson. 2005. survival estimates and risk factors for failure with 6 × 5.7 mm implants. *Int. J. Oral Maxillofac. Implants* 20(6):930–937.

Rhinelander, F.W. 1974a. Tibial blood supply in relation to fracture healing, *Clin. Orthop.* 105:34.

Rhinelander, F.W. 1974b. The normal circulation of bone and its response to surgical intervention. *J. Biomed. Mater. Res.* 8:87.

Tarnow, D., N. Elian, P. Fletcher, S. Froum, S.C. Cho, M. Salama, H. Salama, and D.A. Garber. 2003. Vertical distance from the crest of bone to the height of the interproximal papilla between adjacent implants. *J. Periodontol.* 74:1785–1788.

Chapter 10 Periodontal Medicine Including Biopsy Techniques

Vikki Noonan, DMD, DMSc, and Sadru Kabani, DMD, MS

GINGIVAL NODULES

Nodular proliferations on the gingiva are frequently encountered and represent a number of distinct entities with different etiologies and treatment strategies. While most represent reactive or inflammatory processes, occasionally lesions arise that are developmental in nature, perhaps resulting from stimulation of residua of odonotogenesis that persist in the oral mucosa following tooth development.

PARULIS

Inflammatory infiltrates at the apices of nonvital teeth occasionally channelize through medullary alveolar bone, penetrate the cortical bone and soft tissue, and drain into the oral cavity. These inflammatory infiltrates typically follow a path of least resistance. Given this trend, in most regions inflammatory apical lesions will drain into the oral cavity through a sinus tract on the buccal aspect of the alveolar bone due to decreased thickness of the buccal cortical plate compared with the lingual cortex. Exceptions to this rule are the mandibular second and third molars, the palatal roots of maxillary molars and the maxillary lateral incisors, which typically perforate lingually. At the orifice of the sinus tract, a focal nodular proliferation of inflamed granulation tissue may arise, termed a "parulis" or "gum boil" (Fig. 10.1).

The parulis represents a focus of communication between a pathologic cavity associated with an odontogenic infection and the oral cavity. Therefore, it is frequently possible to insert a gutta-percha point into the sinus tract and trace its path to the tooth that represents the source of the infection. If the sinus tract remains patent, chronic drainage will allow the offending tooth to be asymptomatic. If the sinus tract becomes obstructed, symptoms of odontogenic infection will typically arise. A parulis typically resolves following endodontic therapy or extraction of the offending tooth; however, residual microorganisms and inflammation that persist along a sinus tract following treatment may cause the parulis to persist. In such instances, excision may be required.

FIBROMA

A fibroma represents a nodular proliferation of dense fibrous connective tissue that arises secondary to trauma or focal irritation. Representing the most common reactive proliferation of the oral cavity, fibromas typically present as smooth-surfaced firm nodular lesions that are similar in color to the surrounding mucosa (Fig. 10.2). If the lesion is frequently traumatized or subjected to constant irritation, surface ulceration or hyperkeratosis may result. One form of fibroma with distinctive clinicopathologic characteristics termed the *giant cell fibroma* appears to have no association with trauma and is often described clinically as having a papillary surface architecture. With a predilection for occurring on the gingiva (Magnusson and Rasmusson 1995), the giant cell fibroma is typically diagnosed in patients under age 30. The histopathologic appearance is distinctive due to the presence of multinucleated and stellate cells throughout the densely collagenized connective tissue stroma thought to be derived from

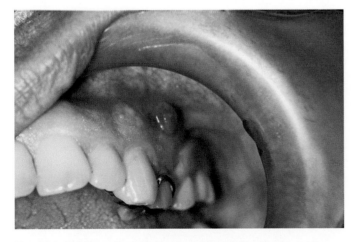

Fig. 10.1 Nodular erythematous mass of granulation tissue near the mucobuccal fold and associated with an asymptomatic nonvital premolar. (Image courtesy of Dr. Helen Santis.)

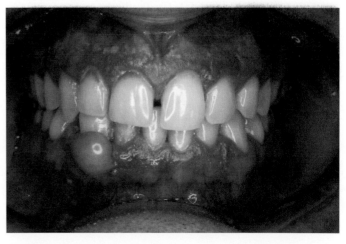

Fig. 10.2 Pink, smooth-surfaced nodular mass of the mandibular attached gingiva. (Image courtesy of Dr. Helen Santis.)

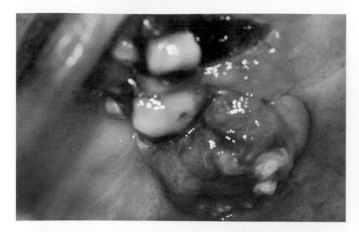

Fig. 10.3 Erythematous ulcerated mass of the palatal gingiva.

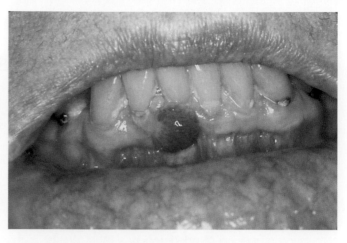

Fig. 10.4 Erythematous nodular mass arising from the mandibular anterior gingiva.

the fibroblast lineage (Souza et al. 2004); however, the presence of these stellate and multinucleated fibroblasts in this lesion is of no known clinical significance.

PERIPHERAL OSSIFYING FIBROMA

Representing a reactive nodular proliferation of fibrous and mineralized tissue, the peripheral ossifying fibroma is a frequently encountered lesion arising exclusively on the gingiva, most often from the region of the maxillary interdental papilla (Fig. 10.3). More common in females, the lesion typically presents in young patients anterior to the first molars (Cuisia and Brannon 2001) and may exhibit surface ulceration (Buchner and Hansen 1979). Although the pathogenesis is not completely understood, the peripheral ossifying fibroma is thought to represent a reactive process that frequently arises secondary to local irritation.

PYOGENIC GRANULOMA

The pyogenic granuloma represents an acquired vascular lesion of the skin and mucous membranes that occurs in patients over a wide age range. Clinically presenting as a nodular lesion remarkable for rapid growth and frequently exhibiting surface ulceration, the pyogenic granuloma often bleeds on subtle provocation secondary to its vascular nature. Pyogenic granulomas of the oral cavity most commonly present on the gingiva in areas of focal chronic irritation (Fig. 10.4).

These lesions have been reported to occur with greater frequency in pregnant women. This increased incidence is likely related to increased levels of estrogen and progesterone, which have been shown to enhance angiogenesis in traumatized tissues (Yuan et al. 2002).

PERIPHERAL GIANT CELL GRANULOMA

Arising exclusively on the gingiva, the peripheral giant cell granuloma presents as an exophytic sessile or pedunculated nodular lesion that is often dark red or purple. Although seen over a wide age range, the peripheral giant cell granuloma typically presents during the fifth to sixth decades of life, is more commonly encountered in females, and is seen with greater frequency in the mandible anterior to the first molars (Bodner et al. 1997, Buduneli et al. 2001) (Fig. 10.5). Focal irritation is typically deemed the causative agent rather than a true neoplastic process. At least one study suggests diminished salivary flow rate and altered salivary composition may increase susceptibility to such lesions due to reduced ability to clear local irritants (Bodner et al. 1997). A pressure resorptive defect of the underlying bone may be appreciated in association with the peripheral giant cell granuloma having a "scooped-out" radiolucent appearance.

DIAGNOSIS AND TREATMENT OF REACTIVE GINGIVAL NODULES

Treatment of reactive gingival nodules, including the gingival fibroma, the peripheral ossifying fibroma, pyogenic granuloma, and peripheral giant cell granuloma, includes both a thorough excision of lesional tissue and removal of local irritants such as calculus or overextended restorations. Despite a diligent effort at complete excision, the recurrence rate for these lesions approaches 20% (Buduneli et al. 2001, Carrera Grano et al. 2001, Walters et al. 2001). To reduce the likelihood of recurrence, some suggest that reactive gingival lesions be excised to bone. In lesions recalcitrant to treatment, a wider excision including periosteum and curettage of the periodontal ligament may be indicated to prevent recurrence (Buduneli et al. 2001, Carrera Grano et al. 2001, Walters et al. 2001).

GINGIVAL CYST OF THE ADULT

The gingival cyst of the adult represents an infrequently encountered lesion of odontogenic origin. Thought to originate from rests of dental lamina, the gingival cyst of the adult pre-

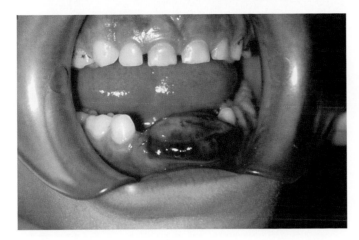

Fig. 10.5 Ulcerated reddish-purple mass of the mandibular anterior gingiva.

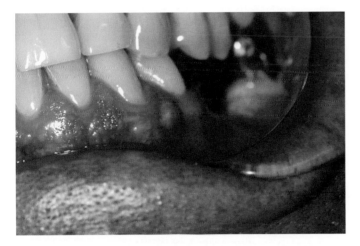

Fig. 10.6 Fluid-filled lesion in the mandibular premolar region of the attached gingiva.

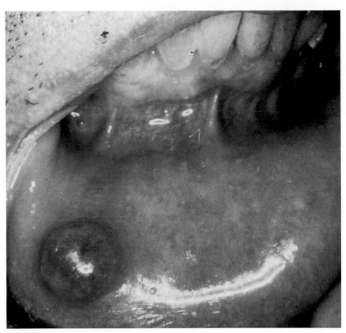

Fig. 10.7 Bluish fluctuant swelling of the lower labial mucosa. (Image courtesy of Dr. Helen Santis.)

sents as a fluid-filled swelling typically arising on the labial attached gingiva of the premolar-canine region of the mandible (Buchner and Hansen 1979, Nxumalo and Shear 1992) (Fig. 10.6). Reported to primarily present during the fifth and sixth decades of life (Giunta 2002, Nxumalo and Shear 1992), the gingival cyst of the adult may occasionally cause a pressure resorptive defect of the subjacent alveolar bone that may cause the entity to be mistaken for a lateral periodontal cyst (Giunta 2002). Rare examples of multiple lesions have been described (Giunta 2002, Shade et al. 1987). Treatment consists of simple surgical excision with submission of lesional tissue for histopathologic examination.

MUCOCELE

The mucocele is a frequently encountered lesion of the oral mucosa characterized by extravasated mucoid material that

leads to a fluctuant nodular swelling of the mucosa, often remarkable for a bluish hue. Typically found on the lower labial mucosa lateral to the midline (Fig. 10.7) but noted in the buccal mucosa, floor of the mouth (ranula), and the anterior ventral tongue, mucoceles frequently arise secondary to a focal traumatic injury that causes rupture of an excretory duct with subsequent spillage of mucin into the surrounding connective tissue. The feeder salivary gland typically retains its capacity to produce secretion; however, the damaged duct prevents passage of saliva into the oral cavity. Patients typically complain of the lesion waxing and waning as the gland produces saliva and then empties. Occasionally, mucoceles are found on the posterior palate, posterior buccal mucosa, and retromolar trigone; most frequently, these lesions represent superficial mucoceles. These lesions typically present as small fluid-filled vesicles that rupture, leaving ulcerative lesions that occasionally recur. Tarter control toothpaste (Navazesh 1995) has been linked to the formation of these lesions, and they have also been described to occur more frequently at mealtime.

Additionally, superficial mucoceles have been reported in early stages of graft-versus-host disease (Garcia et al. 2002). A *mucous cyst* represents a true cystic lesion; the lining is derived from salivary ductal epithelium. These lesions are frequently located in the lips and buccal mucosa and are seen in association with ductal obstruction such as sialolithiasis that may increase intraluminal pressure; however, true developmental cystic lesions are seen.

DESQUAMATIVE GINGIVITIS

Desquamative gingivitis is a clinically descriptive term that is characterized by sloughing, erythematous areas of the attached gingiva. These desquamative gingival changes may be appreciated in the context of vesiculoerosive conditions, including pemphigus vulgaris, mucous membrane (cicatricial) pemphigoid, erosive lichen planus, linear IgA disease, graft-versus-host disease, paraneoplastic pemphigus, epidermolysis bullosa acquisita, systemic lupus erythematosus, chronic ulcerative stomatitis, contact hypersensitivity reactions, and foreign-body gingivitis (2003) (Portions reprinted with permission from the Journal of the Massachusetts Dental Society 2005 Fall;54(3):38).

LICHEN PLANUS

Lichen planus represents an immunologically mediated mucocutaneous disease that affects the oral cavity in as much as 2% of the population. Typically presenting in the fourth to fifth decades of life, lichen planus is characterized by a variety of clinical manifestations including the reticular, erosive, and atrophic forms of the disease. The most commonly affected site is the buccal mucosa, followed by the tongue, gingiva, labial mucosa and lower labial vermilion (Eisen 2002). In just under 10% of patients lichen planus presents exclusively on the gingiva (Eisen 2002, Mignogna et al. 2005) (Fig. 10.8). These cases typically present as the reticular or erosive forms of the disease involving wide areas of marginal and attached gingiva and most commonly affect women (Mignogna et al. 2005). A number of medications (especially antihypertensive agents), flavoring agents, oral hygiene products, and candies and chewing gum can elicit a mucosal reaction clinically indistinguishable from lichen planus. Termed *lichenoid mucositis,* clinical features, when correlated with histopathologic findings, help to distinguish the entity from bona fide lichen planus (Thornhill et al. 2006). Diagnosis is based on a process of elimination of suspected stimuli. This is frequently based on trial and error and is time consuming. If there is a reason to suspect medication-induced mucositis, consultation with the patient's physician may be helpful to explore the possibility of substituting the medication. It is reasonable to treat this affliction with topical corticosteroids to control symptoms. *Chronic ulcerative stomatitis* represents an infrequently encountered condition that shares clinical features of erosive lichen planus superficially and may present as desquamative gingivitis. While the tongue and buccal mucosa are more commonly affected, gingival involvement is clinically indistinguishable from the erosive form of lichen planus (Solomon et al. 2003). This condition typically presents in women and is characterized by episodes of waxing and waning. Differences in the immunofluorescence profile aid in distinguishing chronic ulcerative stomatitis from lichen planus. The immunopathologic pattern for lichen planus is nonspecific but frequently consists of shaggy deposition of fibrinogen along the epithelial–connective tissue interface, whereas that of chronic ulcerative stomatitis consists of IgG

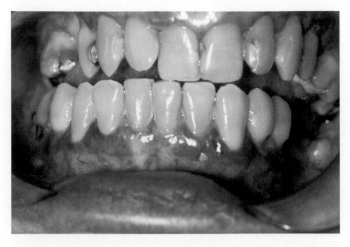

Fig. 10.8 Erosive lichen planus presenting as desquamative gingivitis with erythema and discomfort. (Image courtesy of Dr. Helen Santis.)

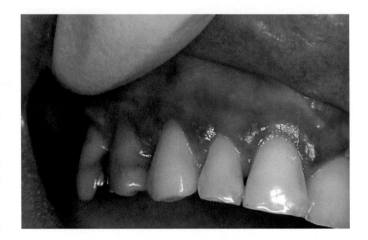

Fig. 10.9 Focal areas of painful erythematous marginal gingiva.

autoantibodies directed against parabasal and basal stratified squamous epithelial cell nuclei. In some instances, a lichenoid appearance of the gingiva is seen secondary to the impregnation of dental materials into the gingiva during dental treatment. The term *foreign body gingivitis* is used to describe this entity. More common in females, foreign body gingivitis typically presents as an erythroplakic or erythroleukoplakic lesion of the gingiva (Fig. 10.9) that does not respond to improved oral hygiene measures or minimal improvement with topical steroid therapy as a result of its anti-inflammatory effect (Gordon 2000).

PEMPHIGUS VULGARIS

Pemphigus vulgaris represents an autoimmune-mediated mucocutaneous disease characterized by autoantibody attack against components of desmosomes. Frequently representing the initial manifestation of the disease, oral lesions are

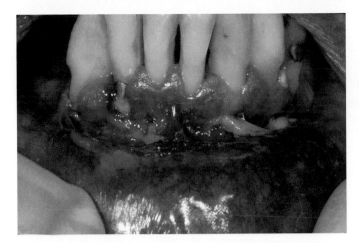

Fig. 10.10 Erosive lesions affecting the anterior mandibular gingiva and mandibular mucobuccal fold.

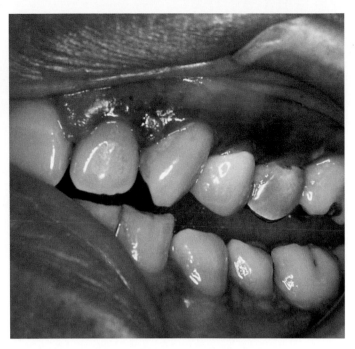

Fig. 10.11 Desquamative gingival lesions representing the only affected site in this patient. (Image courtesy of Dr. Helen Santis.)

found in most instances and typically present as blisters or erosive lesions of the oral and pharyngeal mucosa. Often the onset is insidious with lesions getting progressively worse over time. Desquamative gingivitis in absence of other clinical features is a frequently encountered clinical presentation. Here, blisters and/or erosive lesions are seen often extending to the free gingival tissues (Mignogna et al. 2001) (Fig. 10.10). Direct immunofluorescence findings from tissue submitted in Michel's media shows IgG or IgM antibodies and complement (typically C3) deposited in the intercellular areas of the epithelium. A condition linked to underlying lymphoproliferative disease termed *paraneoplastic pemphigus* may present with oral mucosal involvement yielding clinical characteristics indistinguishable from pemphigus vulgaris. In this condition, circulating autoantibodies produced in response to lymphoid neoplasia crossreact with antigens associated with epithelial desmoplakins and desmosomal proteins. Involvement of the oral mucosa is frequently seen and has been reported as the only manifestation of the disease (Bialy-Golan et al. 1996, Wakahara et al. 2005). Clinically, painful oral erosions and blister formation are appreciated on any mucosal surface including the labial vermilion. Skin eruptions are typically seen. Direct immunofluorescence findings for paraneoplastic pemphigus show deposition of IgG and complement intercellularly within the epithelium and in a linear fashion along the basement membrane. These findings together with a history of lymphoproliferative disease and unique circulating autoantibody profile help to distinguish paraneoplastic pemphigus from other vesiculobullous disorders.

MUCOUS MEMBRANE (CICATRICIAL) PEMPHIGOID

Mucous membrane (cicatricial) pemphigoid represents a group of immune-mediated mucocutaneous disorders in which autoantibodies are directed against basement membrane components. Although the disease typically affects patients in the fifth to sixth decades of life, rare examples of pemphigoid have presented in childhood; in some instances, lesions were limited exclusively to the gingiva (Cheng et al. 2001, Laskaris et al. 1988, Musa et al. 2002, Sklavounou and Laskaris 1990) (Fig. 10.11). Characterized by subepithelial separation from the underlying connective tissue, cicatricial pemphigoid presents as areas of erosive or vesiculobullous change throughout the oral mucosa with subsequent scarring. Ocular involvement and conjunctival scarring caused by the disease can lead to blindness. A subgroup of patients more severely affected by the disease appear to have both IgG and IgA circulating anti–basement membrane zone antibodies and frequently require systemic management (Setterfield et al. 1998). One condition clinically indistinguishable from cicatricial pemphigoid termed *linear IgA disease* is characterized by deposition of IgA along the basement membrane. The immunostaining profile is distinct from that of cicatricial pemphigoid, which is characterized by liner deposition of IgG (and occasionally IgM and IgA) and C3 along the basement membrane and is used to distinguish the two disease processes.

DIAGNOSIS AND TREATMENT OF DESQUAMATIVE GINGIVAL LESIONS

Nonspecific inflammation frequently obscures critical features of underlying disease; therefore, it is recommended to avoid marginal gingiva when choosing a biopsy site for the diagnosis of mucosal fragility disorders. Prior to biopsy, verification of epithelial fragility should be sought by assessing the presence of the Nikolsky sign. Here, firm lateral pressure along the mucosal surface of clinically unremarkable tissue adjacent to involved mucosa will elicit bulla formation. Specimens representing the surface of a "de-roofed" vesicle may occasionally yield useful diagnostic information; therefore, any tissue obtained from clinical manipulation of the friable mucosa should be submitted for immunofluorescence analysis (Siegel and Anhalt 1993); however, a biopsy of perilesional tissue is recommended for diagnostic purposes. The specimen should be bisected with half and submitted in formalin for routine hematoxylin and eosin staining, and the other half should be submitted in immunofluorescence medium such as Michel's for direct immunofluorescence. Immunofluorescence staining in conjunction with light microscopy is often required to make a definitive diagnosis of vesiculobullous disorders (Gallagher et al. 2005). Treatment of symptomatic lichen planus should begin after biopsy and histopathologic diagnosis. In mild cases, topical corticosteroids (0.05% fluocinonide gel [Lidex]) applied to the affected areas sparingly 4 times a day typically provides improvement in the symptoms and clinical appearance of the lesions within 4 weeks. For the most successful management, the patient is instructed to eat, brush, and then apply the gel with nothing per mouth for 30 minutes. It is important that the patient understands this is not a "cure" but rather an effort to maintain remission. More severe cases may require a brief course of systemic corticosteroid therapy in close consultation with the patient's physician. Once the patient is in remission, the patient can be maintained with topical steroids. With the use of topical or systemic corticosteroids, it is not uncommon for patients to develop superimposed candidiasis. A 1-week course of fluconazole (Diflucan) 100-mg tablets (two tablets the first day and then one tablet each day following for 2 weeks) should provide relief in the absence of contraindications. In lesions consistent with foreign-body gingivitis, surgical excision of affected tissue is typically the requisite treatment approach. (Gravitis et al. 2005). In some instances, it is possible to identify the source of the foreign material using energy-dispersive x-ray microanalysis (Daley and Wysocki 1990, Gordon 1997, 2000). Chronic ulcerative stomatitis is frequently recalcitrant to topical steroid therapy and may require management with hydroxychloroquine (Plaquenil) 200 mg/day; however, systemic side effects, including irreversible retinopathy, neuromyopathy, agranulocytosis, aplastic anemia, and toxic psychosis (Solomon et al. 2003), associated with this medication necessitates consultation with a patient's physician and close clinical follow-up. The management of pemphigus vulgaris and mucous membrane pemphigoid typically involves use of systemic corticosteroid therapy; however, a contemporary management approach involves treatment with Rituximab and intravenous immune globulin (Ahmed et al. 2006). It is necessary to have patients evaluated by a physician knowledgeable about this contemporary approach to management.

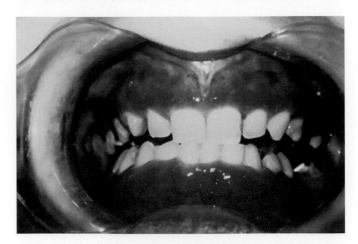

Fig. 10.12 Diffuse, erythematous changes of the attached and free gingival tissues.

PLASMA CELL GINGIVITIS

Plasma cell gingivitis represents a unique entity characterized by sharply demarcated erythema and enlargement of the free and attached gingiva (Fig. 10.12). This condition generally represents a hypersensitivity reaction to flavoring agents in oral hygiene products, candies or chewing gum, medications, or a component of the diet (Macleod and Ellis 1989, Serio et al. 1991). Despite this fact, in many instances the offending antigen cannot be isolated. Biopsies of such lesions show a dense infiltrate of plasma cells within the connective tissue stroma subjacent to the epithelium. Because a neoplastic plasma cell proliferation cannot always be excluded on light microscopic examination alone, additional studies to determine the nature of the infiltrate may be indicated. In cases of idiopathic plasma cell gingivitis or cases representing a hypersensitivity reaction, the plasma cell infiltrate is polyclonal and does not show an atypical profile on immunoelectrophoresis. When other oral mucosal sites are involved, the condition is termed *plasma cell mucositis.* Here, diffuse, erythematous, and edematous changes may involve multiple areas of the oral mucosa (Heinemann et al. 2006, Kaur et al. 2001). Treatment of plasma cell gingivomucositis requires that the patient record all food intake and eliminate possible dietary culprits. Additionally, discontinuance of use of chewing gums, candies, and/oral hygiene products remarkable for strong flavoring agents such as peppermint or cinnamon should be encouraged. Unfortunately, in some instances the underlying causative agent cannot be identified. Topical steroid agents (fluocinonide 0.05% gel [Lidex]) applied to the affected areas sparingly 4 times a day may provide some improvement. This regimen is most effective if the patient eats, brushes, and then applies the gel to the affected areas with nothing per mouth for 30 minutes following application. It is generally recommended that follow up evaluation after 4 weeks of topical corticosteroid application be done and the frequency of use adjusted until improvement is optimal.

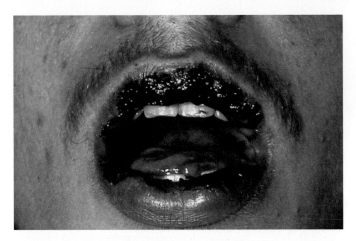

Fig. 10.13 Ulceration and crusting lesions involving the labial vermilion.

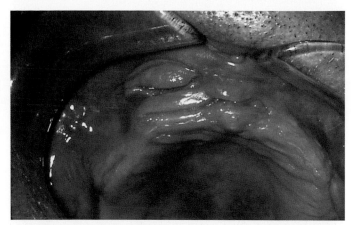

Fig. 10.14 Redundant hyperplastic folds of tissue in the anterior maxillary associated with a maxillary denture.

ERYTHEMA MULTIFORME

Representing an acute hypersensitivity reaction involving the skin and the mucosa, erythema multiforme (EM) most typically presents in the third and fourth decades of life; however, a significant number of patients diagnosed with EM are children (Huff et al. 1983, Wine et al. 2006). Although the pathogenesis is poorly understood, the condition is likely an immune-mediated disorder. EM is induced by a variety of factors, of which the most common include bacterial and viral infectious agents and medications, most typically analgesics and antibiotics. Approximately 50% of cases arise subsequent to infection with herpes simplex virus. Two forms of EM are typically described: erythema multiforme major and erythema multiforme minor. EM minor presents with lesions involving the skin and/oral mucosa. It is often recurrent, with the most frequent cause of recurrent EM being a herpes simplex virus infection (Huff et al. 1983, Sinha et al. 2006). EM major is also referred to as *Stevens Johnson syndrome* and is typically triggered by mycobacterium and medications (Huff et al. 1983). Here, in addition to cutaneous and/oral lesions, ocular and/or genital mucosae are affected. Symblephara or bands of scar tissue within the conjunctiva can lead to blindness akin to ocular lesions of cicatricial pemphigoid. The most severe form of EM termed *toxic epidermal necrolysis* (Lyell's disease) involves sloughing and ulceration of large areas of the skin and mucosa. Mucosal lesions of EM are characterized by painful ulcerative lesions of acute onset (Fig. 10.13), often involving the labial mucosa with crusting of the vermilion. Gingival involvement is rare but is occasionally reported. Classic skin eruptions are described as "target lesions" and are seen in approximately 25% of all patients presenting with EM (Ayangco and Rogers 2003). Here, concentric erythematous rings likened in appearance to a target or "bull's eye" are appreciated on the extremities initially and occasionally extending to involve other cutaneous sites. Unlike other vesiculobullous disorders, the attached mucosae including that of the gingiva and hard palate are typically unaffected by the process. In most instances, EM resolves spontaneously over the course of a 2- to 4-week period. Treatment is typically supportive and directed at managing symptoms. In severe cases one may consider systemic corticosteroid therapy. Here, prednisone tablets (10 mg) may be prescribed with the instruction to take 6 tablets in the morning until the lesions recede and then decrease by 1 tablet on each successive day (Arm et al. 2001). Dexamethasone (Decadron) elixir 0.5 mg/5 mL can also be used. Here, one can recommend the patient rinse with 1 tablespoonful (15 mL) for 3 days 4 times per day and swallow. Then, for 3 days, rinse with 1 teaspoonful (5 mL) 4 times a day and swallow. Then, for 3 days, rinse with 1 teaspoonful (5 mL) 4 times a day and swallow every other time. Last, the patient should rinse with 1 teaspoonful (5 mL) 4 times per day and expectorate (Arm et al. 2001). If recurrent EM is thought to be precipitated by herpes simplex virus, antiviral medications are typically prescribed such as systemic acyclovir (Zovirax) 400 mg capsules administering 1 tablet 3 times daily or valacyclovir (Valtrex) 500-mg capsules administering 1 tablet per day.

GINGIVAL ENLARGEMENT

Gingival enlargement may be focal or diffuse in nature. Focal gingival enlargement is seen in association with a number of entities ranging from benign reactive proliferations to malignant epithelial neoplasia. Generalized gingival enlargement is likewise seen in association with a variety of conditions. Systemic medications, neoplastic infiltration, infection, and hereditary conditions may all present with generalized gingival enlargement. The diagnosis and treatment of such lesions are discussed later.

EPULIS FISSURATUM

Epulis fissuratum is characterized by folds of hyperplastic fibrovascular connective tissue that develop in association with an ill-fitting denture. These redundant folds of tissue frequently extend into the vestibule with invaginations to accommodate the denture flange (Fig. 10.14). Treatment consists of surgical

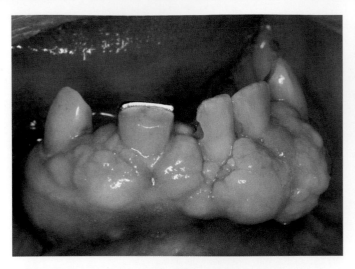

Fig. 10.15 Marked gingival hyperplasia in a patient using calcium channel blocker agents.

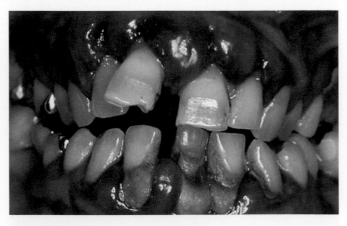

Fig. 10.16 Diffuse enlargement and erythema of the marginal and papillary gingiva.

excision to ensure improved soft tissue contour for impression making and fabrication of a new prosthesis.

MEDICATION-INDUCED GINGIVAL OVERGROWTH

Numerous medications have been implicated as the causative agent for diffuse gingival enlargement. The medications most commonly associated with gingival overgrowth include calcium channel blockers (Fig. 10.15), cyclosporine, and anticonvulsant medications. Although incompletely understood, it seems such medications target a common pathway of collagen degradation; interference with this pathway induces fibrosis and extracellular matrix overgrowth in the gingival tissues (Kataoka et al. 2005, McCulloch 2004). Introduction of the causative medication in childhood seems to increase the likelihood of occurrence. The most typical clinical course for the process begins as diffuse gingival enlargement of the facial surfaces of the gingiva most prominently along the interdental papillae several weeks following the initiation of a medication. Over time, the tissue overgrowth extends to the lingual surfaces of the gingiva and can completely cover the dentition. Typically, hyperplastic changes are not appreciated in edentulous areas unless the tissues approximate poorly fitting prostheses or surround dental implants. Oral hygiene dictates the clinical appearance of the hyperplastic gingival tissues. In patients with adequate oral hygiene, the hyperplastic tissues maintain a pink color and stippled appearance. In patients with marginal oral hygiene, the tissues may become friable and bleed on subtle provocation.

Treatment for medication-induced gingival hyperplasia includes substitution of the inciting medication with a different agent that is less likely to cause gingival hyperplasia when possible and encouraging meticulous oral hygiene. Additionally, supplementation with folic acid may reduce the incidence of medication-induced gingival overgrowth; however, the results of such efforts have been mixed (Backman et al. 1989, Brown et al. 1991, Drew et al. 1987, Prasad et al. 2004). Azithromycin has been shown to significantly reduce gingival overgrowth in patients taking cyclosporine (Tokgoz et al. 2004). In some instances, however, surgical intervention is indicated. Although a variety of surgical techniques may be used, such as gingivectomy or flap surgery, laser excision with submission of lesional tissue for histopathologic examination has been shown to represent a favorable method of management (Mavrogiannis et al. 2006).

HYPERPLASTIC GINGIVITIS

Diffuse erythematous enlargement of the gingival tissues is frequently seen secondary to poor oral hygiene (Fig. 10.16). Diabetes mellitus (Mealey 2006) and smoking have also been implicated in the development of hyperplastic gingivitis. Treatment requires professional scaling and curettage and improved oral hygiene measures. Chemopreventive measures such as 0.12% chlorhexidine rinse may be used if debridement and improved oral hygiene measures alone do not provide resolution. Surgical recontouring of the gingival tissues using a scalpel or laser may be indicated for patients who are recalcitrant to conservative treatment.

LEUKEMIA

Leukemia represents a hematopoietic stem cell malignancy that produces a number of clinical signs and symptoms intimately associated with a proliferation of atypical leukocytes and subsequent reduced numbers of normal circulating leukocytes and erythrocytes. The most typical oral lesions associated with leukemia include ulcerative lesions, spontaneous gingival bleeding, and gingival hyperplasia (Weckx et al. 1990) (Fig. 10.17). In many instances, oral lesions represent the first sign of the disease. The systemic signs and symptoms of leukemia are numerous and include malaise,

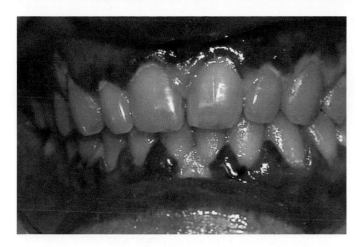

Fig. 10.17 Diffuse gingival enlargement and hemorrhage in this patient subsequently diagnosed with monocytic leukemia.

fever, fatigue, and lymphadenopathy. Gingiva ranks among the most common sites of extramedullary disease (Wiernik et al. 1996) and is most typically involved in patients with acute myeloid leukemia, particularly the subtypes of acute monocytic and myelomonocytic leukemia. Diffuse gingival enlargement characterized by a boggy consistency with spontaneous bleeding or bleeding on subtle provocation should be viewed with a high index of suspicion. A scalpel biopsy with submission of lesional tissue for histopathologic and immunohistochemical analysis is indicated.

GINGIVAL FIBROMATOSIS

Gingival fibromatosis represents a disorder characterized by progressive enlargement of gingival tissues secondary to increased numbers of collagen fiber bundles. While gingival fibromatosis may be idiopathic, it is often hereditary, with most cases showing autosomal dominant inheritance. While most cases represent isolated examples of the disorder, gingival fibromatosis is also seen in association with a number of hereditary syndromes. In addition to functional concerns such as difficulty eating, speaking, and maintaining oral hygiene, gingival fibromatosis causes aesthetic concerns for the patient. Gingival fibromatosis is characterized by painless diffuse gingival enlargement of normal color and firm, fibrous consistency with minimal bleeding (Coletta and Graner 2006). Typically arising at the time of primary or permanent tooth eruption, gingival fibromatosis frequently causes malpositioning of teeth, retention of primary dentition, delayed eruption of the permanent dentition, and other functional and esthetic concerns.

Treatment traditionally involves gingivectomy using serial gingival resections together with strict oral hygiene measures. One recent report suggests a more aggressive surgical protocol of gingivectomy, odontectomy, and alveolar ridge os-

tectomy of an entire arch at a time eliminates recurrence (Odessey et al. 2006); however, the management strategy employed depends on the individual case and wishes of the patient.

LIGNEOUS GINGIVITIS AND CONJUNCTIVITIS

Ligneous gingivitis represents a rare disorder characterized by deposition of amyloid-like material within the gingival connective tissue subjacent to the oral mucosa. Ligneous conjunctivitis is frequently seen in association with gingival lesions and represents an autosomal recessive form of chronic membranous conjunctivitis (Bateman et al. 1986). Many cases of ligneous conjunctivitis are related to plasminogen deficiency and present in patients of Turkish origin (Gokbuget et al. 1997, Gunhan et al. 1999). It is hypothesized that plasminogen deficiency caused inability of fibrinolytic activity to clear fibrin deposits, allowing accumulation of this material. Clinical presentation can include gingival enlargement with multiple areas of ulceration involving both arches (Scully et al. 2001), a change that mimics gingival enlargement associated with leukemia. At least one case of ligneous gingivitis affecting the alveolar mucosa in the absence of conjunctivitis in a patient without plasminogen deficiency has been reported (Naudi et al. 2006). The best management strategy for these lesions at the present is uncertain. In individuals with plasminogen deficiency, intravenous purified plasminogen concentrate has been used (Schott et al. 1998); however, this therapy is not widely available.

WEGENER'S GRANULOMATOSIS

Wegener's granulomatosis represents a necrotizing granulomatous vasculitis most commonly involving the respiratory tract and kidneys. Oral lesions have been described and are characterized by gingival hyperplasia remarkable for a rough, granular appearance often likened to that of a strawberry and bleed with subtle provocation (Manchanda et al. 2003). Isolated gingival lesions may represent the initial manifestation of the disease in approximately 7% of patients (Patten and Tomecki 1993) and begin initially in the interdental papilla spreading to the adjacent gingival tissues. In one case report, the disease initially presented as a poorly healing extraction socket in a young patient (Kemp et al. 2005). Other oral lesions may also be present, including mucosal ulcerations, nodular lesions of the labial mucosa, and palatal osteonecrosis. Biopsy with confirmation using antinuclear cytoplasmic antibody (ANCA) testing is critical. It is important to include Wegener's granulomatosis in a differential diagnosis of gingival hyperplasia, particularly in a patient with a history of sinusitis, given the poor prognosis associated with the condition if left untreated.

PIGMENTED LESIONS

Pigmented lesions are encountered with some frequency in the oral cavity. In some instances, these lesions represent

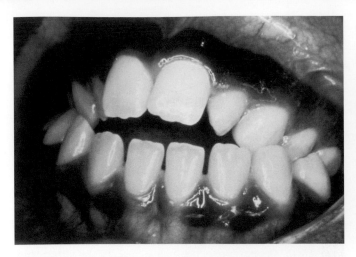

Fig. 10.18 Band-like pigmentation of the attached gingiva. (Image courtesy of Dr. Helen Santis.)

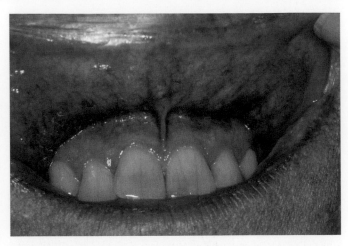

Fig. 10.19 Pigmentation of the gingiva associated with use of minocycline.

generalized or diffuse changes; in other instances, the pigmented change is focal in nature.

PHYSIOLOGIC PIGMENTATION

Most commonly noted on attached gingiva in darker-skinned patients, physiologic pigmentation presents as a diffuse brown-black pigmentation secondary to increased melanocyte activity. Here, pigmentation develops during the first two decades of life. Physiologic pigmentation is typically bilaterally symmetrical in distribution and most prominent along the labial attached gingiva in the region of the maxillary and mandibular incisors. The distribution is likened to a ribbon-like band that spares the marginal gingiva (Eisen 2000) (Fig. 10.18). Pigmentation may also be appreciated within the buccal mucosa, lips, tongue (particularly of the fungiform papillae), and hard palate and is notable for a macular appearance with indistinct borders (Kauzman et al. 2004). Although physiologic pigmentation is not a medical concern, recent publications suggest social pressures influence some patients to request gingival depigmentation for esthetic purposes (Tal et al, Oegiesser and Ta. 2003). The most significant factor for clinicians is to recognize the entity as a normal manifestation as opposed to a pathologic process.

MEDICATION-INDUCED PIGMENTATION

Drug-induced discoloration of the oral mucosa is caused by an increasing number of medications. The discoloration can occur after direct contact with the medication or following its systemic absorption. In some instances, medication stimulates melanocytes to increase melanin production; in other instances, medication causes formation of metabolites that are thought to be the cause of increased pigmentation. Medications typically associated with pigmentation of the oral mucosa include minocycline (Fig. 10.19), antimalarial medications, estrogens, tranquilizers, phenolphthalein found in

laxatives, chemotherapy medications, and medications used to manage patients with HIV infection (Abdollahi and Radfar 2003). In some instances, discoloration caused by medication resolves in the weeks following discontinuation of the medication; however, in some instances, the change is permanent. Many accounts of exposure to metals such as gold, lead, mercury, and silver have been historically documented in the literature with a classic presentation of linear pigmentation following the gingival margins described. Other presentations of drug-induced pigmentation vary but include diffuse pigmentation of the palate and rare descriptions of pigmentation changes of the soft tissues of the lips, tongue, eyes, and perioral skin.

Antimalarial agents are typically linked to discoloration of the palate; minocycline use is frequently associated with palatal and occasionally skin lesions (Treister et al. 2004); phenolphthalein is associated with well-circumscribed macular pigmented lesions of the skin and mucosa; and estrogens are associated with diffuse melanosis and most typically seen in female patients. In some instances, a biopsy may be indicated to confirm the diagnosis and rule out the presence of underlying melanocytic pathology.

SMOKER'S MELANOSIS

Smoker's melanosis represents diffuse benign pigmentation of the oral mucosa, particularly noted on the anterior facial attached gingiva (Axell and Hedin 1982, Hedin 1977) (Fig. 10.20). Typically, the distribution of pigmented changes begins in the interdental papilla region and may extend to form continuous ribbons involving the anterior attached gingiva with the apical extension of the lesions not exceeding the mucogingival junction (Hedin 1977). Unlike physiologic pigmentation, smoker's melanosis does not spare the marginal gingiva, is of recent onset, and increases in intensity and number of lesions

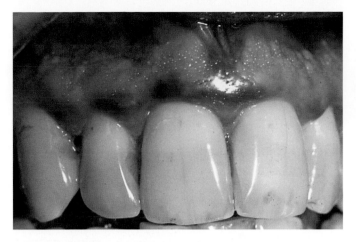

Fig. 10.20 Diffuse pigmentation of the anterior attached gingiva in a heavy smoker. (Image courtesy of Dr. Brad Neville.)

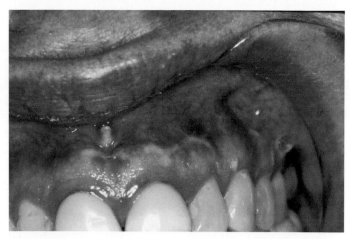

Fig. 10.21 Multifocal areas of mucosal pigmentation at the apices of teeth treated with apical retrofill procedures. (Image courtesy of Dr. Helen Santis.)

with an increase in the number of cigarettes used daily. In patients who consume alcohol in addition to smoking, areas of oral depigmentation surrounded by hyperpigmentation are frequently noted (Natali et al. 1991). In a study of dark-skinned patients, while most non–tobacco users exhibited some level of physiologic oral melanin pigmentation, tobacco smokers had significantly more oral surfaces pigmented than did the non–tobacco users (Ramer and Burakoff 1997). Reports have been described of reduction in smoking leading to the disappearance of smoking-induced melanosis (Hedin et al. 1993). Given that these lesions present in patients in adulthood and often darken progressively over time, biopsy is often indicated to rule out melanoma. (Portions reprinted with permission from the Journal of the Massachusetts Dental Society 2007 Spring;in press).

AMALGAM TATTOO

An amalgam tattoo typically presents as a gray-blue macular lesion of the oral mucosa that occurs following implantation of dental amalgam into the oral soft tissues (Fig. 10.21). Common clinical scenarios associated with this phenomenon include introduction of amalgam into the oral soft tissues by high-speed hand pieces, contamination of extraction sites with amalgam debris, and linear impregnation of interdental tissues with amalgam-laden dental floss following restorative procedures (Mirowski and Waibel 2002). Small radiopaque particles may be evident on radiographic examination to corroborate the clinical impression; however, the metallic particles are often too small to be appreciated. Over time, an amalgam tattoo may appear to enlarge as the amalgam-carrying macrophages migrate away from the initial site of implantation. In some individuals, an inflammatory response to the amalgam may be accompanied by clinical discomfort that would predicate the need for biopsy. When a suspected amalgam tattoo presents in an unusual location, a biopsy

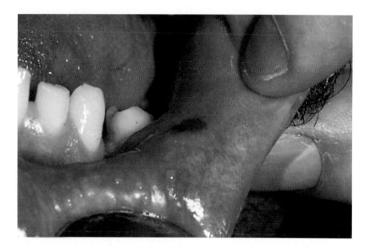

Fig. 10.22 Well-demarcated brown macular lesion of the lower labial mucosa.

may be indicated to exclude other pigmented lesions such as melanoacanthoma and melanoma. (Portions reprinted with permission from the Journal of the Massachusetts Dental Society 2005 Spring;54(1):55).

MELANOTIC MACULE

The oral melanotic macule is a frequently encountered pigmented lesion of the oral mucosa. Typically found on the lower labial vermilion, buccal mucosa, gingiva, and palate, the oral melanotic macule is characterized as a solitary, well-demarcated, uniformly pigmented, macular brown lesion (Fig. 10.22). Although exposure to ultraviolet radiation can clearly be excluded as a causative agent in intraoral lesions, the relationship between lesions of the lower labial vermillion and sun exposure is unclear. While the oral melanotic macule is

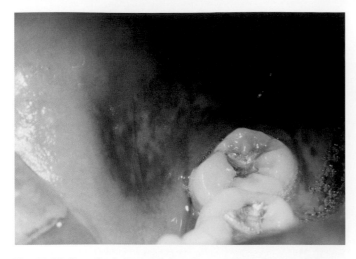

Fig. 10.23 Smooth pigmented lesion of recent onset of the posterior buccal mucosa.

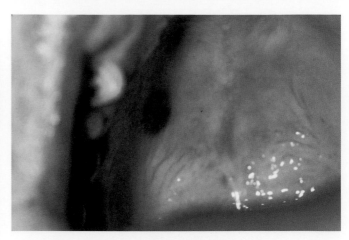

Fig. 10.24 Slightly raised pigmented lesion of the posterior hard palate.

generally not regarded as a lesion with potential to undergo malignant transformation, rare examples of malignant transformation have been reported in the literature (Kahn et al. 2005). Given the predilection for melanoma to present on the gingiva and palate, lesions presenting in these locations should be viewed with a high index of suspicion. Additionally, features such as asymmetry and color variegation are worrisome. Because malignancy cannot always be excluded on clinical presentation alone, an excisional biopsy may be indicated with submission of lesional tissue for histopathologic evaluation.

ORAL MELANOACANTHOMA (MELANOACANTHOSIS)

Oral melanoacanthoma represents an acquired melanocytic pigmentation that arises suddenly and most likely represents a reactive phenomenon. Presenting most frequently in black females, the lesion is characterized by a brown-black appearance exhibiting a smooth to somewhat raised surface contour (Fig. 10.23). Typically found on the buccal mucosa, oral melanoacanthoma has been reported to arise on the lip, palate, and gingiva (Flaitz 2000). As the lesion arises suddenly with marked growth potential, melanoacanthoma cannot be differentiated from other melanocytic lesions without biopsy. Distinctive histopathologic features particularly the presence of dendritic melanocytes within the epithelial spinous cell layer differentiates melanoacanthoma from other melanocytic lesions. Once definitive diagnosis is made, further treatment is unnecessary. Although rare, cases of spontaneous resolution of oral melanoacanthoma have been reported (Fatahzadeh and Sirois 2002, Wright 1988).

ORAL MELANOCYTIC NEVUS

Oral melanocytic nevi typically present as well-circumscribed papules that range in color from brown to black and may be devoid of pigmentation (Fig. 10.24). The most common locations for melanocytic nevi in the oral cavity include the buccal mucosa, gingiva, lips, and palate (Buchner and Hansen 1987, 1987). One form of melanocytic nevus termed the *blue nevus* typically presents on the palate (Buchner and Hansen 1987, 1987). Oral melanocytic nevi are somewhat more common in women and occur over a wide age range, with most lesions noted in the third to fourth decades of life (Buchner et al. 2004). Although the malignant transformation potential of oral mucosal melanoma is not proved, given that oral melanocytic nevi frequently present on the palate, similar to oral mucosal melanoma, and are relatively uncommon lesions, excision with submission of lesional tissue for histopathologic evaluation is recommended.

ORAL MELANOMA

Typically occurring on the palate, maxillary gingiva, and maxillary alveolar mucosa (Barker et al. 1997), oral melanoma represents an uncommon malignancy of the oral cavity. The 5-year survival rate for oral melanoma persists unchanged since initially being reported in the literature and ranges from 10% to 20% (Eisen and Voorhees 1991). Oral melanoma presents as pigmented plaques remarkable for irregular asymmetric borders exhibiting brown-black coloration (Fig. 10.25). Some melanomas are notable for lack of melanocytic pigmentation (Eisen and Voorhees 1991). Clinical evidence of ulceration, bone erosion, or frank invasion of bone is not uncommon. When intraoral melanoma represents metastatic rather than a primary oral lesion, such lesions typically present on the buccal mucosa, tongue, and at the site of a nonhealing extraction socket (Patton et al. 1994). Given that the prognosis of oral melanoma depends on the stage of the disease at the time of diagnosis and that the depth of most oral lesions at the time of diagnosis is advanced, early detection is critical. Pigmented lesions with irregular borders presenting

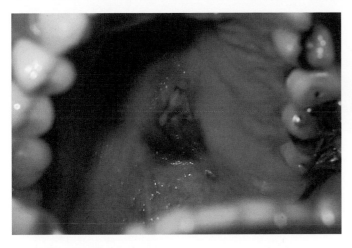

Fig. 10.25 Irregular pigmented lesion of the posterior palate.

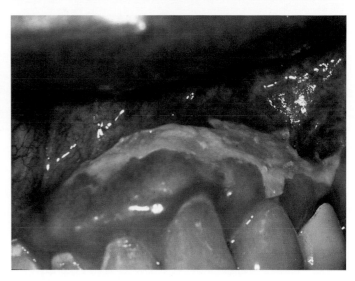

Fig. 10.26 White plaque of the maxillary mucobuccal fold.

on the palate or maxillary gingiva or alveolar mucosa should be viewed with suspicion. Treatment typically involves radical surgical excision together with neck dissection and adjuvant chemotherapy (Umeda and Shimada 1994).

SANGUINARIA-INDUCED LEUKOPLAKIA

Exposure of the oral cavity to chemical substances, medications, or dentifrice can lead to specific mucosal changes. Chronic use of mouth rinses containing sanguinaria extract (also known as bloodroot extract) has been shown to produce leukoplakic lesions with an implied potential for malignant transformation (Damm et al. 1999). The use of Viadent brand mouth rinse (Colgate Oral Pharmaceuticals, Canton, MA) containing sanguinaria extract, a product of the bloodroot plant, has been shown to produce leukoplakic lesions of the maxillary vestibule, a site that is uncommon for white lesions (Fig. 10.26). It is generally recognized that these lesions frequently persist and even recur following discontinuation of the product. Because biopsy may show areas of mild to moderate epithelial dysplasia, these patients need to be kept under close surveillance (Eversole et al. 2000). Given the apparent association between sanguinaria-containing dentifrice and dysplastic leukoplakia, it is recommended individuals presenting with leukoplakic lesions and history of exposure to Viadent submit for biopsy and discontinue use of the product (Damm et al. 1999). (Portions reprinted with permission pending from Otolaryngol Clin N Am (38)2005 21-35).

PROLIFERATIVE VERRUCOUS LEUKOPLAKIA

One particularly persistent and importunate form of leukoplakia can be difficult to distinguish from verrucous carcinoma. Proliferative verrucous leukoplakia (PVL) is characterized as an extensive exophytic papillary proliferation that often involves multiple sites and is recalcitrant to treatment.

Initial PVL lesions present in a solitary fashion characterized by thin hyperkeratosis and are well delineated from the surrounding mucosa. As the lesion evolves, it may develop a perceptually thickened quality with superficial undulations consistent with verrucous hyperplasia. The lesions become multifocal and recur following excision. Over time, the lesions progress to verrucous carcinoma or squamous cell carcinoma (Hansen et al. 1985).

Unique in its predilection for women nearly 4:1 over men, PVL is generally diagnosed in the seventh decade of life. Studies report from 70% to nearly 100% of PVL lesions progress to squamous cell carcinoma (Batsakis et al. 1999, Silverman and Gorsky 1997), with the gingiva and tongue being the sites showing the highest incidence of transformation (Silverman and Gorsky 1997). Months to years may transpire from the time of initial recognition of the process to its ultimate transformation to invasive carcinoma. No apparent link between use of tobacco products has been firmly established with regard to PVL (Fettig et al. 2000, Silverman and Gorsky 1997), and the link between human papilloma virus and PVL is controversial (Bagan et al. 2007, Palefsky et al. 1995). Given that PVL most likely represents a disease that is multifactorial in nature, it is difficult to anticipate specifically who is at high risk for developing the condition. (Portions reprinted with permission pending from Otolaryngol Clin N Am (38)2005 21-35).

MALIGNANT NEOPLASIA

Malignant neoplasia involving the oral cavity may represent primary disease or metastasis, particularly from the breast, lung, kidney, prostate, gastrointestinal tract, and thyroid gland.

SQUAMOUS CELL CARCINOMA

Oral squamous cell carcinoma represents the most common intraoral malignancy and is remarkable for a variety of clinical presentations ranging from erythroplakia to leukoplakia, or it may present as a combination of the two. Incipient lesions are typically painless; however, as the lesion progresses, areas of ulceration and induration may be seen and the lesion may become more nodular. Fixation to underlying tissues and local-regional lymph node metastasis indicate further progression to an intermediate stage of malignancy. Late-stage lesions may present with bony involvement, tooth mobility, pain, and paresthesia (Zakrzewska 1999).

All forms of tobacco use are associated with an increased risk of developing oral squamous cell carcinoma. When combined, tobacco and alcohol work in synergy to potentiate the increased risk of developing invasive tumor (Scully and Porter 2000, Zakrzewska 1999). Additionally, exposure to ultraviolet radiation (lip) or betel quid (a mixture of slaked lime, areca nut, and tobacco wrapped in betel leaf and chewed—a social habit quite prevalent in the Indian subcontinent) may predispose susceptive individuals to submucous fibrosis, a condition that has an approximately 17% chance of malignant transformation and immunosuppression; these are well-recognized etiologic factors that when paired with a genetically susceptible individual may yield transformation to oral squamous cell carcinoma (Scully and Porter 2000).

The most common sites for oral squamous cell carcinoma are the posterior lateral and ventral tongue, floor of the mouth, and soft palate, although gingival lesions are also reported (Seoane et al. 2006) (Fig. 10.27). In some instances, the similarities between gingival squamous cell carcinoma and periodontal disease may lead to a delay in diagnosis. The prognosis for oral squamous cell carcinoma is largely based on the stage of presentation (Sanderson and Ironside 2002) and the lesion's location. The presence of positive nodal involvement reduces long-term survival by as much as 50% (Sanderson and Ironside 2002).

Clinical presentations that warrant immediate action to rule out squamous cell carcinoma include nonhealing ulceration or unexplained swelling of approximately 3 weeks' duration and all red and/or white lesions. A biopsy is mandatory with definitive diagnosis via histolopathologic examination. Additionally, it is recommended that tooth mobility unrelated to periodontal disease receive thorough investigation (Sanderson and Ironside 2002).

Early biopsy is recommended for any nonhealing or slowly resolving lesion even if the patient is young and/or denies exposure to tobacco products. Although extremely rare, occasional accounts of squamous cell carcinoma arising in pediatric patients have been made (Bill et al. 2001). Additionally, recent reports have shown an increased incidence of

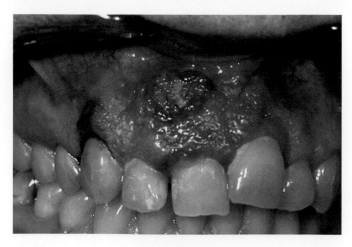

Fig. 10.27 Exophytic erythroleukoplakic lesion of the anterior maxillary gingiva.

squamous cell carcinoma in female patients and in those patients younger than 40 years (Martin-Granizo et al. 1997). Ultimately, despite advances in treatment, prognosis depends heavily on tumor staging at the time of presentation. Thorough clinical examination and a high index of suspicion for mucosal alterations at high-risk sites provide the best chance for a positive outcome. (Portions reprinted with permission pending from Otolaryngol Clin N Am (38)2005 21-35).

VERRUCOUS CARCINOMA

Verrucous carcinoma represents a low-grade variant of squamous cell carcinoma with a characteristic papillary exophytic growth pattern (Fig. 10.28). A superficial insidious neoplasm principally due to its indolent growth course, verrucous carcinoma can be extensive and multifocal at the time of clinical presentation. Within the oral cavity, the most common sites of occurrence are the buccal mucosa and gingiva, sites typically not considered "high risk" with regard to traditional squamous cell carcinoma (Koch et al. 2001).

Although verrucous carcinoma is not confined exclusively in presentation to the upper aerodigestive tract, a significant link between oral verrucous carcinoma and tobacco products has been made (Ferlito and Recher 1980, Medina et al. 1984, Spiro 1998). Surgical excision is advocated as the standard of care for treatment, and many years of follow-up are required to capture additional foci, as dictated by the multicentric nature of the process and apparent increased likelihood that recurrent lesions may prove to be more poorly differentiated than their predecessor (Ferlito and Recher 1980, Medina et al. 1984, Spiro 1998). Further, studies have reported a near 20% incidence of squamous cell carcinoma arising in lesions of verrucous carcinoma. Clinical distinction

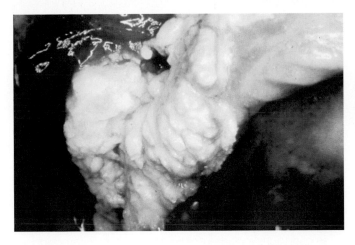

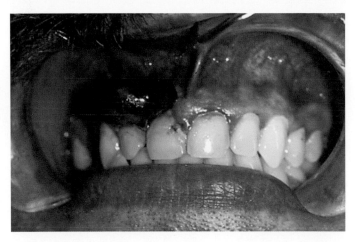

Fig. 10.28 Extensive exophytic white papillary lesion involving the edentulous maxillary alveolar ridge and vestibule.

Fig. 10.29 Metastatic melanoma to the anterior maxillary gingiva.

cannot be made between traditional verrucous carcinoma lesions and those containing foci of invasive squamous cell carcinoma (Medina et al. 1984). This finding dictates thorough surgical excision extending deep into connective tissue to allow adequate assessment of the epithelial–connective tissue interface histologically and that multiple levels through the specimen be subjected to histologic evaluation. Given the propensity for verrucous carcinoma lesions to grow in a slow fashion, adequate surgical excision coupled with rigorous clinical follow-up provides the most optimistic prognosis (McCoy and Waldron 1981). (Portions reprinted with permission pending from Otolaryngol Clin N Am (38)2005 21-35).

METASTATIC DISEASE

Although metastatic disease is uncommon in the oral cavity, representing less than 1% of oral neoplasia (van der Waal et al. 2003), in at least one third of patients, metastasis to the jawbones or oral soft tissues represents the first clinical sign of the disease (D'Silva et al. 2006, Hirshberg and Buchner 1995, van der Waal et al. 2003). Of lesions inclined to metastasize to the oral soft tissues, metastatic disease from the lung is the most commonly encountered (Hirshberg and Buchner 1995). When lesions metastasize to the gingiva, lesions typically present as polypoid masses that may be mistaken for a benign reactive gingival nodule (Ramon Ramirez et al. 2003) (Fig. 10.29), and the most common primary tumors to metastasize to the gingiva are those originating in the lung, kidney, breast, bone, and liver (Elkhoury et al. 2004). Obviously, it is of utmost importance to distinguish metastatic disease from benign lesions that can share similar clinical features. Biopsy with submission of lesional tissue for histopathologic analysis is important to ensure the best prognosis.

INFECTIONS

The oral cavity is susceptible to infections with fungal, bacterial and viral organisms. Infections with herpes simplex virus and/oral manifestations of HIV infection are discussed later.

HERPES

Primary herpetic infection typically presents as gingivostomatitis with the recurrence manifesting as cutaneous/mucocutaneous disease. Symptoms of primary herpetic stomatitis arise after an incubation period of up to 3 weeks following infection. The prodromal symptoms are not pathognomonic and include malaise, fever, headache, nausea, anorexia, and irritability. Acute onset of pain in the oral cavity is seen with the development of numerous small vesicular lesions that quickly coalesce and ulcerate. These lesions may involve any area of the oral cavity, including the gingiva, buccal mucosa, tongue, palatal mucosa, vermillion, perioral skin, and oropharynx. A severe complication of primary herpetic gingivostomatitis is ocular involvement. After initial infection, oral herpes simplex virus remains latent in the trigeminal ganglion. Upon activation, the virus utilizes the axons of sensory neurons as a means to reach overlying tissues. Symptomatic recurrences are common and can be preceded by a prodrome of "tingling" or discomfort in the affected region, sometimes initially mistaken for a toothache. The typical clinical presentation for recurrent intraoral herpetic infection is of multiple "punched-out" painful areas of ulceration that may coalesce and often follow the distribution of the greater palatine nerve. Recurrences are frequently attributed to manipulation of oral tissues during routine dental procedures. The distinction between recurrent herpetic lesions and recurrent apthous stomatitis (canker sores) is that herpetic ulcerations

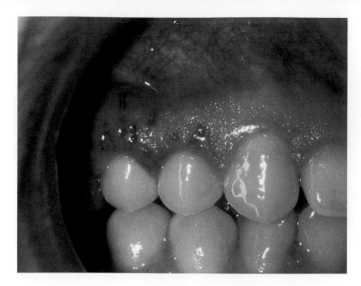

Fig. 10.30 Multiple painful punctate areas of ulceration involving the maxillary attached gingiva.

typically involve keratinized tissues (Fig. 10.30) and recurrent apthous ulcerations are seen on moveable mucosa. Systemic antiviral therapy is generally accepted as being effective for management of primary herpetic stomatitis using acyclovir (Zovirax) 200-mg capsules administering 1 capsule 5 times a day for 5 to 7 days; however, the effectiveness of other antiviral medications such as famciclovir or valaciclovir has not been fully evaluated (Arduino and Porter 2006). Further, the optimal timing of initiating therapy and optimum dose are not fully defined. Reduction of clinical signs and patient symptoms has been reported for recurrent herpetic stomatitis using acyclovir (Zovirax) cream (5%) one application topically every 3 to 4 hours for 5 days and penciclovir (Denavir) cream (1%) every 2 hours for 5 days, but studies are still needed to determine which is more effective (Arduino and Porter 2006). A recent report advocates the utility of oral famciclovir (Famvir) in the management of herpes labialis (Spruance et al. 2006). Here, 1500 mg is taken within 1 hour of the onset of prodromal symptoms. This protocol was reported to reduce duration of symptoms by approximately 2 days. In immunocompromised patients, topical therapeutics offer little benefit. Acyclovir remains the medication of choice (Arduino and Porter 2006). As self-inoculation is possible, it is recommended patients be advised to avoid touching the lesions and then touching the eyes, genitalia, or other body areas to prevent infection at new sites. (Portions reprinted with permission from the Journal of the Massachusetts Dental Society 2005 Winter; 53(4):55).

HIV-ASSOCIATED GINGIVITIS

Initially termed "HIV-related gingivitis," linear gingival erythema presents as a red band involving the free gingival mar-

gin. This change is typically most prominent in the region of the anterior dentition but extends to involve the posterior quadrants with some frequency (Reznik 2005). Mild bleeding on subtle provocation has been reported, and efforts at improved oral hygiene do not lead to resolution. Some reports suggest this pattern of gingivitis represents a form of candidiasis (Velegraki et al. 1999). Lesions typically resolve following professional plaque removal and rinses with a 0.12% suspension of chlorhexidine gluconate twice per day for 2 weeks. Additional HIV-related conditions involving the gingiva include *necrotizing ulcerative gingivitis* (NUG) involving necrosis of one or more interdental papillae and *necrotizing ulcerative periodontitis* with features of NUG in addition to rapidly progressing loss of periodontal attachment. Treatment for these conditions includes gentle debridement with povidone-iodine irrigation. The standard management approach includes rinsing with a suspension of 0.12% chlorhexidine. Follow-up with additional debridement at 24 hours and again every 7 to 10 days is required. In the acute phase with systemic symptoms of fever and malaise, antibiotic therapy is indicated (amoxicillin 2 g a day for 7 days or metronidazole).

ORAL SOFT TISSUE BIOPSY TECHNIQUES

It is usually prudent to recommend a biopsy on lesions that have persisted for over 2 weeks after the removal of a potential irritant. Lesions that are related to infection, inflammation, or local trauma may resolve during this time.

Biopsies can be incisional or excisional depending on the nature of the lesion and the comfort level and skills of the practitioner. If the lesion is large or malignancy is suspected, an incisional biopsy is indicated in order to not compromise the definitive treatment of the potentially malignant lesion. If the lesion is benign, located away from vital structures and of small diameter (less than 1 cm), an excisional biopsy could be recommended. In both cases, it is important to include some of the surrounding healthy tissue in the biopsy specimen. The incision should be made parallel to the normal course of nerves, arteries, and veins to minimize injury (Ellis 2003). Also, when opting for an incisional biopsy you should keep in mind that "deeper is better" and it is much better to take a deep, narrow biopsy rather than a broad, shallow one in order to not miss the cellular changes at the base of the lesion (Ellis 2003). Because of the size and morphology of the lesion requiring an incisional approach, it is sometimes necessary to obtain more than one biopsy sample of the same lesion (different locations).

The following methods are used to collect tissue samples from the oral cavity (Campisi et al. 2003, Ellis 2003).
- Needle biopsy

- Tissue punch biopsy

- Scalpel biopsy

- Laser biopsy

This chapter will be limited to describing techniques using scalpel biopsy.

ARMAMENTARIUM

Surgical set that is recommended is given in *Practical Periodontal Plastic Surgery* (Dibart and Karima).

INCISIONAL SCALPEL BIOPSY

After proper local anesthesia is achieved by infiltrating the area 1 cm peripheral to the lesion with xylocaine 2% with 1:100,000 epinephrine, the surgeon focuses on the area where the incision will take place. With a No. 15 blade, a small wedge that is approximately 3 mm deep, 5 mm long, and 3 mm wide is excised. The specimen needs to include a portion of the margin as well as some healthy tissue. The specimen is then very delicately transferred to a biopsy container with 10% formalin. It is very important not to crush the tissues during excision or transfer into the fixative solution as that may interfere with the proper oral pathology diagnosis. The surgical site can be closed with a single suture; the patient is given some mild analgesics (acetaminophen 500 mg) and advised to rinse with an antiseptic mouthwash (chlorhexidine 0.12%) for 1 week.

EXCISIONAL SCALPEL BIOPSY

After proper local anesthesia is achieved by infiltrating the area 1 cm peripheral to the lesion with xylocaine 2% with 1:100,000 epinephrine, an elliptical incision is made around the lesion with the blade angled toward the lesion (Fig. 10.31). Tissue stabilization and hemostasis can be achieved manually (assistant's fingers pinching the soft tissue on both sides of the biopsy) or mechanically by using a clamp (i.e., Chalazion clamp for a biopsy of the lip) (Fig. 10.32). Again, it is important to remember to remove some healthy tissue with the specimen. The rule of thumb for easy closure is to have an ellipse that is 3 times longer than wide. Also, depending on the location of the biopsy site and the size of the wound, there may be a need to undermine the mucosa (with scissors) in order to obtain tension-free closure. Primary closure of an elliptic wound is easily achieved provided that the margins of the wound are gently undermined.

Elliptical incisions on the attached gingiva or palate are not sutured but are left to heal by secondary intention. The excised specimen is then very delicately transferred to a biopsy container with 10% formalin for fixation (Fig. 10.33). Again, it is very critical not to crush the tissues during excision or transfer into the fixative solution as that may interfere with the proper oral pathology diagnosis.

The patient is given some mild analgesics (acetaminophen 500 mg) and advised to rinse with an antiseptic mouthwash (chlorhexidine 0.12%) for 1 week.

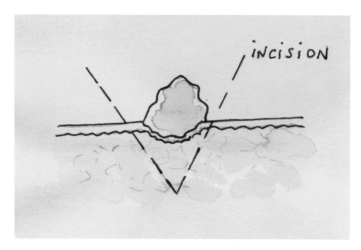

Fig. 10.31 Excisional biopsy. Notice the angulation of the blade, which will create a wedge as well as the amount of healthy tissue removed.

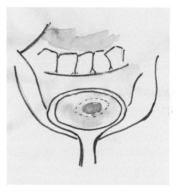

Fig. 10.32 Elliptical incision to remove a growth located on the lower lip. The lip is stabilized here with a Chalazion clamp.

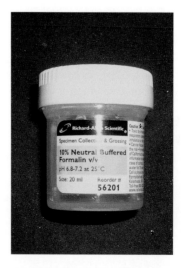

Fig. 10.33 Biopsy container, the amount of liquid present should be sufficient to completely cover the biopsy specimen.

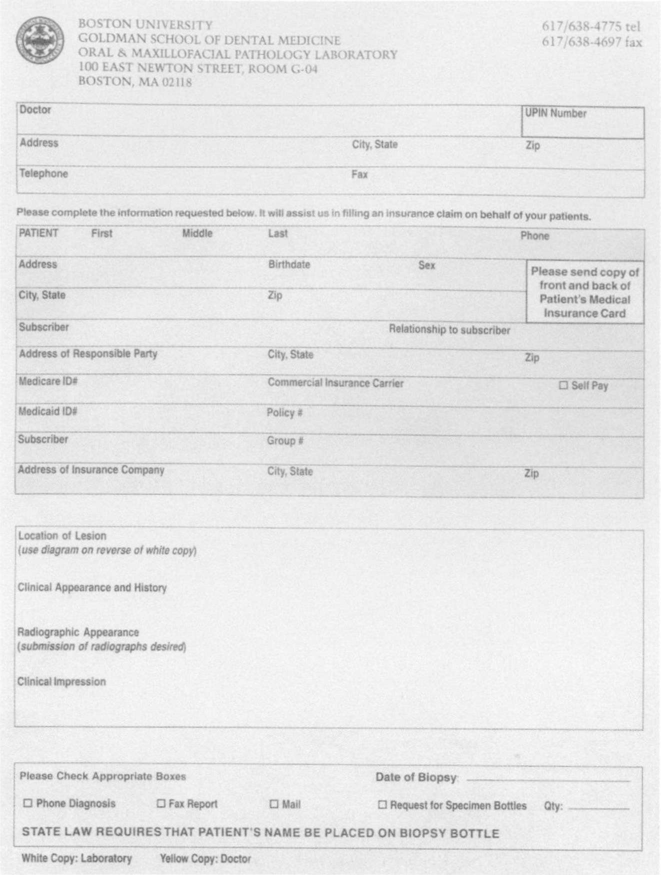

BOSTON UNIVERSITY
GOLDMAN SCHOOL OF DENTAL MEDICINE
ORAL & MAXILLOFACIAL PATHOLOGY LABORATORY
100 EAST NEWTON STREET, ROOM G-04
BOSTON, MA 02118

617/638-4775 tel
617/638-4697 fax

Doctor | UPIN Number

Address | City, State | Zip

Telephone | Fax

Please complete the information requested below. It will assist us in filling an insurance claim on behalf of your patients.

PATIENT First Middle Last | Phone

Address | Birthdate | Sex

City, State | Zip

Please send copy of front and back of Patient's Medical Insurance Card

Subscriber | Relationship to subscriber

Address of Responsible Party | City, State | Zip

Medicare ID# | Commercial Insurance Carrier | ☐ Self Pay

Medicaid ID# | Policy #

Subscriber | Group #

Address of Insurance Company | City, State | Zip

Location of Lesion
(use diagram on reverse of white copy)

Clinical Appearance and History

Radiographic Appearance
(submission of radiographs desired)

Clinical Impression

Please Check Appropriate Boxes | Date of Biopsy:
☐ Phone Diagnosis ☐ Fax Report ☐ Mail ☐ Request for Specimen Bottles Qty:
STATE LAW REQUIRES THAT PATIENT'S NAME BE PLACED ON BIOPSY BOTTLE

White Copy: Laboratory   Yellow Copy: Doctor

Fig. 10.34 Biopsy Data Sheet used at Boston University School of Dental Medicine, Oral and Maxillofacial Pathology Laboratory.

BIOPSY DATA SHEET

Once the specimen has been placed in formalin and the patient discharged, the biopsy data sheet must be completed in its entirety. Patient's information including age and gender as well as the lesion's size, location of the biopsy, and a clinical diagnosis are typically required (Fig. 10.34). This sheet must accompany the biopsy container and must be sent to the oral pathology laboratory without delay.

REFERENCES

Anonymous. 1987. The histomorphologic spectrum of peripheral ossifying fibroma. *Oral Surg. Oral Med. Oral Pathol.* 63(4):452-461.

Anonymous. 1987. Pigmented nevi of the oral mucosa: a clinicopathologic study of 36 new cases and review of 155 cases from the literature. Part I: a clinicopathologic study of 36 new cases. *Oral Surg. Oral Med. Oral Pathol.* 63(5):566-572.

Anonymous. 1987. Pigmented nevi of the oral mucosa: a clinicopathologic study of 36 new cases and review of 155 cases from the literature. Part II: analysis of 191 cases. *Oral Surg. Oral Med. Oral Pathol.* 63(6):676-682.

Anonymous. 2002. The clinical features, malignant potential, and systemic associations of oral lichen planus: a study of 723 patients. *J. Am. Acad. Dermatol.* 46(2):207-214.

Anonymous. 2003. Position paper: oral features of mucocutaneous disorders. *J. Periodontol.* 74(10):1545-1556.

Abdollahi, M., and M. Radfar. 2003. A review of drug-induced oral reactions. *J. Contemp. Dent. Pract.* 4(1):10-31.

Ahmed, A.R., Z. Spigelman, L.A. Cavacini, and M.R. Posner. 2006. Treatment of pemphigus vulgaris with rituximab and intravenous immune globulin. *N. Engl. J. Med.* 355(17):1772-1779.

Arduino, P.G., and S.R. Porter. 2006. Oral and perioral herpes simplex virus type 1 (HSV-1) infection: review of its management. *Oral Dis.* 12(3):254-270.

Arm, R.N., et al. 2001. In M.A. Siegel, S. Silverman Jr., and T.P. Sollecito, editors. *Clinician's Guide to Treatment of Common Oral Conditions,* 5th ed. BC Decker, New York.

Axell, T., and C.A. Hedin. 1982. Epidemiologic study of excessive oral melanin pigmentation with special reference to the influence of tobacco habits. *Scand. J. Dent. Res.* 90(6):434-442.

Ayangco, L., and R.S. Rogers 3rd. 2003. Oral manifestations of erythema multiforme. *Dermatol. Clin.* 21(1):195-205.

Backman, N., A.K. Holm, L. Hanstrom, H.K. Blomquist, J. Heijbel, and G. Safstrom. 1989. Folate treatment of diphenylhydantoin-induced gingival hyperplasia. *Scand. J. Dent. Res.* 97(3):222-232.

Bagan, J.V., Y. Jimenez, J. Murillo, C. Galvada, R. Poveda, C. Scully, T.M. Alberola, M. Torres-Puente, and M. Perez-Alonso. 2007. Lack of association between proliferative verrucous leukoplakia and human papillomavirus infection. *J. Oral Maxillofac. Surg.* 46-49.

Barker, B.F., W.M. Carpenter, T.E. Daniels, M.A. Kahn, A.S. Leider, F. Lozada-Nur, D.P. Lynch, R. Melrose, P. Merrell, T. Morton, E. Peters, J.A. Regezi, S.D. Richards, G.M. Rick, M.D. Rohrer, L. Slater, J.C. Stewart, C.E. Tomich, R.A. Vickers, N.K. Wood, and S.K. Young. 1997. Oral mucosal melanomas: the WESTOP Banff workshop proceedings. Western Society of Teachers of Oral Pathology. *Oral Surg. Oral Med. Oral Pathol. Oral Radiol. Endod.* 83(6):672-679.

Bateman, J.B., T.H. Pettit, S.J. Isenberg, and K.B. Simons. 1986. Ligneous conjunctivitis: an autosomal recessive disorder. *J. Pediatr. Ophthalmol. Strabismus* 23(3):137-140.

Batsakis, J.G., P. Suarez, and A.K. el-Naggar. 1999. Proliferative verrucous leukoplakia and its related lesions. *Oral Oncol.* 35(4):354-359.

Bialy-Golan, A., S. Brenner, and G.J. Anhalt. 1996. Paraneoplastic pemphigus: oral involvement as the sole manifestation. *Acta Dermatol. Venereol.* 76(3):253-254.

Bill, T.J., V.R. Reddy, K.L. Ries, T.J. Gampper, and M.A. Hoard. 2001. Adolescent gingival squamous cell carcinoma: report of a case and review of the literature. *Oral Surg. Oral Med. Oral Pathol. Oral Radiol. Endod.* 91(6):682-685.

Bodner, L., M. Peist, A. Gatot, and D.M. Fliss. 1997. Growth potential of peripheral giant cell granuloma. *Oral Surg. Oral Med. Oral Pathol. Oral Radiol. Endod.* 83(5):548-551.

Brown, R.S., P.T. Di Stanislao, W.T. Beaver, and W.K. Bottomley. 1991. The administration of folic acid to institutionalized epileptic adults with phenytoin-induced gingival hyperplasia. A double-blind, randomized, placebo-controlled, parallel study. *Oral Surg. Oral Med. Oral Pathol.* 71(5):565-568.

Buchner, A., and L.S. Hansen. 1979. The histomorphologic spectrum of the gingival cyst in the adult. *Oral Surg. Oral Med. Oral Pathol.* 48(6):532-539.

Buchner, A., P.W. Merrell, and W.M. Carpenter. 2004. Relative frequency of solitary melanocytic lesions of the oral mucosa. *J. Oral Pathol. Med.* 33(9):550-557.

Buduneli, E., N. Buduneli, and T. Unal. 2001. Long-term follow-up of peripheral ossifying fibroma: report of three cases. *Periodontal. Clin. Investig.* 23(1):11-14.

Campisi, G., O. Di Fede, and C. Di Liberto. 2003. [Incisional biopsy in oral medicine: punch vs traditional procedure]. *Minerva Stomatol.* 52(11-12):481-488.

Carrera Grano, I., L. Berini Aytes, and C.G. Escoda. 2001. Peripheral ossifying fibroma. Report of a case and review of the literature. *Med. Oral* 6(2):135-141.

Cheng, Y.S., T.D. Rees, J.M. Wright, and J.M. Plemons. 2001. Childhood oral pemphigoid: a case report and review of the literature. *J. Oral Pathol. Med.* 30(6):372-377.

Coletta, R.D., and E. Graner. 2006. Hereditary gingival fibromatosis: a systematic review. *J Periodontol.* 77(5):753-764.

Culsia, Z.E., and R.B. Brannon. 2001. Peripheral ossifying fibroma—a clinical evaluation of 134 pediatric cases. *Pediatr. Dent.* 23(3):245-248.

Daley, T.D., and G.P. Wysocki. 1990. Foreign body gingivitis: an iatrogenic disease? *Oral Surg. Oral Med. Oral Pathol.* 69(6):708-712.

Damm, D.D., A. Curran, D.K. White, and J.F. Drummond. 1999. Leukoplakia of the maxillary vestibule—an association with Viadent? *Oral Surg. Oral Med. Oral Pathol. Oral Radiol. Endod.* 87(1):61-66.

Dibart, S., and M. Karima. 2006. *Practical Periodontal Plastic Surgery.* Blackwell Publishing, Ames, IA.

Drew, H.J., R.I. Vogel, W. Molofsky, H. Baker, and O. Frank. 1987. Effect of folate on phenytoin hyperplasia. *J. Clin. Periodontol.* 14(6):350-356.

D'Silva, N.J., D.J. Summerlin, K.G. Cordell, R.A. Abdelsayed, C.E. Tomich, C.T. Hanks, D. Fear, and S. Meyrowitz. 2006. Metastatic tumors in the jaws: a retrospective study of 114 cases. *J. Am. Dent. Assoc.* 137(12):1667-1672.

Eisen, D. 2000. Disorders of pigmentation in the oral cavity. *Clin. Dermatol.* 18(5):579-587.

Eisen, D., and J.J. Voorhees. 1991. Oral melanoma and other pigmented lesions of the oral cavity. *J. Am. Acad. Dermatol.* 24(4):527-537.

Elkhoury, J., D.A. Cacchillo, D.N. Tatakis, J.R. Kalmar, C.M. Allen, and P.P. Sedghizadeh. 2004. Undifferentiated malignant neoplasm involving the interdental gingiva: a case report. *J. Periodontol.* 75(9): 1295-1299.

Ellis, E. 2003. Principles of differential diagnosis and biopsy. In L.J. Peterson, E. Ellis III, J.R. Hupp, and M.R. Tucker, editors. *Contemporary Oral and Maxillofacial Surgery*, 4th ed. Elsevier, Philadelphia, pp. 458-478.

Eversole, L.R., G.M. Eversole, and J. Kopcik. 2000. Sanguinaria-associated oral leukoplakia: comparison with other benign and dysplastic leukoplakic lesions. *Oral Surg. Oral Med. Oral Pathol. Oral Radiol. Endod.* 89(4):455-464.

Fatahzadeh, M., and D.A. Sirois. 2002. Multiple intraoral melanoacanthomas: a case report with unusual findings. *Oral Surg. Oral Med. Oral Pathol. Oral Radiol. Endod.* 94(1):54-56.

Ferlito, A., and G. Recher. 1980. Ackerman's tumor (verrucous carcinoma) of the larynx: a clinicopathologic study of 77 cases. *Cancer* 46(7):1617-1630.

Fettig, A., M.A. Pogrel, S. Silverman, Jr., T.E. Bramanti, M. Da Costa, and J.A. Regezi. 2000. Proliferative verrucous leukoplakia of the gingiva. *Oral Surg. Oral Med. Oral Pathol. Oral Radiol. Endod.* 90(6):723-730.

Flaitz, C.M. 2000. Oral melanoacanthoma of the attached gingiva. *Am. J. Dent.* 13(3):162.

Gallagher, G., S. Kabani, and V. Noonan. 2005. Desquamative gingivitis. *J. Mass. Dent. Soc.* 54(3):38.

Garcia, F.V.M.J., M. Pascual-Lopez, M. Elices, E. Dauden, A. Garcia-Diez, and J. Fraga. 2002. Superficial mucoceles and lichenoid graft versus host disease: report of three cases. *Acta Derm. Venereol.* 82(6):453-455.

Giunta, J.L. 2002. Gingival cysts in the adult. *J. Periodontol.* 73(7):827-831.

Gokbuget, A.Y., S. Mutlu, C. Scully, A. Efeoglu, S.R. Porter, P. Speight, G. Erseven, and M. Karacorlu. 1997. Amyloidaceous ulcerated gingival hyperplasia: a newly described entity related to ligneous conjunctivitis. *J. Oral. Pathol. Med.* 26(2):100-104.

Gordon, S. 2000. Foreign body gingivitis associated with a new crown: EDX analysis and review of the literature. *Oper. Dent.* 25(4):344-348.

Gordon, S.C., and T.D. Daley. 1997. Foreign body gingivitis: identification of the foreign material by energy-dispersive x-ray microanalysis. *Oral Surg. Oral Med. Oral Pathol. Oral Radiol. Endod.* 83(5):571-576.

Gravitis, K., T.D. Daley, and M.A. Lochhead. 2005. Management of patients with foreign body gingivitis: report of 2 cases with histologic findings. *J. Can. Dent. Assoc.* 71(2):105-109.

Gunhan, O., M. Gunhan, E. Berker, C.A. Gurgan, and H. Yildirim. 1999. Destructive membranous periodontal disease (Ligneous periodontitis). *J. Periodontol.* 70(8):919-925.

Hansen, L.S., J.A. Olson, and S. Silverman Jr. 1985. Proliferative verrucous leukoplakia. A long-term study of thirty patients. *Oral Surg. Oral Med. Oral Pathol.* 60(3):285-298.

Hedin, C.A. 1977. Smoker's melanosis. *Arch. Dermatol.* 113:1533-1538.

Hedin, C.A., J.J. Pindborg, and T. Axell. 1993. Disappearance of smoker's melanosis after reducing smoking. *J Oral Pathol Med* 22(5):228-230.

Heinemann, C., T. Fischer, U. Barta, A. Michaelides, and P. Elsner. 2006. Plasma cell mucositis with oral and genital involvement—successful treatment with topical cyclosporin. *J. Eur. Acad. Dermatol. Venereol.* 20(6):739-740.

Hirshberg, A., and A. Buchner. 1995. Metastatic tumours to the oral region. An overview. *Eur. J. Cancer B Oral Oncol.* 31B(6):355-360.

Huff, J.C., W.L. Weston, and M.G. Tonnesen. 1983. Erythema multiforme: a critical review of characteristics, diagnostic criteria, and causes. *J. Am. Acad. Dermatol.* 8(6):763-775.

Kahn, M.A., D.R. Weathers, and J.G. Hoffman. 2005. Transformation of a benign oral pigmentation to primary oral melanoma. *Oral Surg. Oral Med. Oral Pathol. Oral Radiol. Endod.* 100(4):454-459.

Kataoka, M., J. Kido, Y. Shinohara, and T. Nagata. 2005. Drug-induced gingival overgrowth—a review. *Biol. Pharm. Bull.* 28(10):1817-1821.

Kaur, C., G.P. Thami, R. Sarkar, and A.J. Kanwar. 2001. Plasma cell mucositis. *J. Eur. Acad. Dermatol. Venereol.* 15(6):566-567.

Kauzman, A., M. Pavone, N. Blanas, and G. Bradley. 2004. Pigmented lesions of the oral cavity: review, differential diagnosis, and case presentations. *J. Can. Dent. Assoc.* 70(10):682-683.

Kemp, S., G. Gallagher, and S. Kabani. 2005. Case report: Oral involvement as an early manifestation of Wegener's granulomatosis. *Oral Surg. Oral Med. Oral Pathol.* 100(2):*187*.

Koch, B.B., D.K. Trask, H.T. Hoffman, L.H. Karnell, R.A. Robinson, W. Zhen, and H.R. Menck. 2001. National survey of head and neck verrucous carcinoma: patterns of presentation, care, and outcome. *Cancer* 92(1):110-120.

Laskaris, G., A. Triantafyllou, and P. Economopoulou. 1988. Gingival manifestations of childhood cicatricial pemphigoid. *Oral Surg. Oral Med. Oral Pathol.* 66(3):349-352.

Macleod, R.I., and J.E. Ellis. 1989. Plasma cell gingivitis related to the use of herbal toothpaste. *Br. Dent. J.* 166(10):375-376.

Magnusson, B.C., and L.G. Rasmusson. 1995. The giant cell fibroma. A review of 103 cases with immunohistochemical findings. *Acta Odontol. Scand.* 53(5):293-296.

Manchanda, Y., T. Tejasvi, R. Handa, and M. Ramam. 2003. Strawberry gingiva: a distinctive sign in Wegener's granulomatosis. *J. Am. Acad. Dermatol.* 49(2):335-337.

Martin-Granizo, R., F. Rodriguez-Campo, L. Naval, and F.J. Diaz Gonzalez. 1997. Squamous cell carcinoma of the oral cavity in patients younger than 40 years. *Otolaryngol Head Neck Surg.* 117 (3 Pt 1):268-275.

Mavrogiannis, M., J.S. Ellis, R.A. Seymour, and J.M. Thomason. 2006. The efficacy of three different surgical techniques in the management of drug-induced gingival overgrowth. *J. Clin. Periodontol.* 33(9): 677-682.

McCoy, J.M., and C.A. Waldron. 1981. Verrucous carcinoma of the oral cavity. A review of forty-nine cases. *Oral Surg. Oral Med. Oral Pathol.* 52(6):623-629.

McCulloch, C.A. 2004. Drug-induced fibrosis: interference with the intracellular collagen degradation pathway. *Curr. Opin. Drug Disc. Dev.* 7(5):720-724.

Mealey, B.L. 2006. Periodontal disease and diabetes: a two-way street. *J. Am. Dent. Assoc.* 137(Suppl 2):26S-31S.

Medina, J.E., W. Dichtel, and M.A. Luna. 1984. Verrucous-squamous carcinomas of the oral cavity. A clinicopathologic study of 104 cases. *Arch. Otolaryngol.* 110(7):437-440.

Mignogna, M.D., L. Lo Muzio, and E. Bucci. 2001. Clinical features of gingival pemphigus vulgaris. *J. Clin. Periodontol.* 28(5):489-493.

Mignogna, M.D., L. Lo Russo, and S. Fedele. 2005. Gingival involvement of oral lichen planus in a series of 700 patients. *J. Clin. Periodontol.* 32(10):1029-1033.

Mirowski, G.W., and J.S. Waibel. 2002. Pigmented lesions of the oral cavity. *Dermatol. Therapy* 15(3):218-228.

Musa, N.J., V. Kumar, L. Humphreys, A. Aguirre, and M.E. Neiders. 2002. Oral pemphigoid masquerading as necrotizing ulcerative gingivitis in a child. *J. Periodontol.* 73(6):657-663.

Natali, C., J.L. Curtis, L. Suarez, and E.J. Millman. 1991. Oral mucosa pigment changes in heavy drinkers and smokers. *J. Natl. Med. Assoc.* 83(5):434-438.

Naudi, K.B., K.D. Hunter, D.G. MacDonald, and D.H. Felix. 2006. Ligneous alveolar gingivitis in the absence of plasminogen deficiency. *J. Oral. Pathol. Med.* 35(10):636-638.

Navazesh, M. 1995. Tartar-control toothpaste as a possible contributory factor in the onset of superficial mucocele: a case report. *Spec. Care Dentist* 15(2):74-78.

Noonan, V., S. Kabani, and G. Gallagher. 2005. Recurrent intraoral herpes infection. *J Mass Dent Soc* 53(4):55.

Nxumalo, T.N., and M. Shear. 1992. Gingival cyst in adults. *J. Oral Pathol. Med.* 21(7):309-313.

Odessey, E.A., A.B. Cohn, F. Casper, and L.S. Schechter. 2006. Hereditary gingival fibromatosis: aggressive 2-stage surgical resection in lieu of traditional therapy. *Ann. Plast. Surg.* 57(5):557-560.

Palefsky, J.M., S. Silverman, Jr., M. Abdel-Salaam, T.E. Daniels, and J.S. Greenspan. 1995. Association between proliferative verrucous leukoplakia and infection with human papillomavirus type 16. *J. Oral Pathol. Med.* 24(5):193-197.

Patten, S.F., and K.J. Tomecki. 1993. Wegener's granulomatosis: cutaneous and/or oral mucosal disease. *J. Am. Acad. Dermatol.* 28 (5 Pt 1):710-718.

Patton, L.L., J.S. Brahim, and A.R. Baker. 1994. Metastatic malignant melanoma of the oral cavity. A retrospective study. *Oral Surg. Oral Med. Oral Pathol.* 78(1):51-56.

Prasad, V.N., H.S. Chawla, A. Goyal, K. Gauba, and P. Singhi. 2004. Folic acid and phenytoin induced gingival overgrowth—is there a preventive effect. *J. Indian Soc. Pedod. Prev. Dent.* 22(2):82-91.

Ramer, M., and R.P. Burakoff. 1997. Smoker's melanosis. Report of a case. *N. Y. State Dent. J.* 63(8):20-21.

Ramon Ramirez, J., J. Seoane, J. Montero, G.C. Esparza Gomez, and R. Cerero. 2003. Isolated gingival metastasis from hepatocellular carcinoma mimicking a pyogenic granuloma. *J. Clin. Periodontol.* 30(10):926-929.

Reznik, D.A. 2005. Oral manifestations of HIV disease. *Top. HIV Med.* 13(5):143-148.

Sanderson, R.J., and J.A. Ironside. 2002. Squamous cell carcinomas of the head and neck. *BMJ* 325(7368):822-827.

Schott, D., C.E. Dempfle, P. Beck, A. Liermann, A. Mohr-Pennert, M. Goldner, P. Mehlem, H. Azuma, V. Schuster, A.M. Mingers, H.P. Schwarz, and M.D. Kramer. 1998. Therapy with a purified plasminogen concentrate in an infant with ligneous conjunctivitis and homozygous plasminogen deficiency. *N. Engl. J. Med.* 339(23):1679-1686.

Scully, C., A.Y. Gokbuget, C. Allen, J.V. Bagan, A. Efeoglu, G. Erseven, C. Flaitz, S. Cintan, T. Hodgson, S.R. Porter, and P. Speight. 2001. Oral lesions indicative of plasminogen deficiency (hypoplasminogenemia). *Oral Surg. Oral Med. Oral Pathol. Oral Radiol. Endod.* 91(3):334-337.

Scully, C., and S. Porter. 2000. ABC of oral health. Oral cancer. *BMJ* 321(7253):97-100.

Seoane, J., P.I. Varela-Centelles, T.F. Walsh, J.L. Lopez-Cedrun, and I. Vazquez. 2006. Gingival squamous cell carcinoma: diagnostic delay or rapid invasion? *J. Periodontol.* 77(7):1229-1233.

Serio, F.G., M.A. Siegel, and B.E. Slade. 1991. Plasma cell gingivitis of unusual origin. A case report. *J. Periodontol.* 62(6):390-393.

Setterfield, J., P.J. Shirlaw, M. Kerr-Muir, S. Neill, B.S. Bhogal, P. Morgan, K. Tilling, S.J. Challacombe, and M.M. Black. 1998. Mucous membrane pemphigoid: a dual circulating antibody response with IgG and IgA signifies a more severe and persistent disease. *Br. J. Dermatol.* 138(4):602-610.

Shade, N.L., W.M. Carpenter, and D.D. Dolzer. 1987. Gingival cyst of the adult. Case report of a bilateral presentation. *J. Periodontol.* 58(11):796-799.

Siegel, M.A., and G.J. Anhalt. 1993. Direct immunofluorescence of detached gingival epithelium for diagnosis of cicatricial pemphigoid. Report of five cases. *Oral Surg. Oral Med. Oral Pathol.* 75(3):296-302.

Silverman, S., Jr., and M. Gorsky. 1997. Proliferative verrucous leukoplakia: a follow-up study of 54 cases. *Oral Surg. Oral Med. Oral Pathol. Oral Radiol. Endod.* 84(2):154-157.

Sinha, A., J. Chander, and S. Natarajan. 2006. Erythema multiforme presenting as chronic oral ulceration due to unrecognised herpes simplex virus infection. *Clin. Exp. Dermatol.* 31(5):737-738.

Sklavounou, A., and G. Laskaris. 1990. Childhood cicatricial pemphigoid with exclusive gingival involvement. *Int. J. Oral Maxillofac. Surg.* 19(4):197-199.

Solomon, L.W., A. Aguirre, M. Neiders, A. Costales-Spindler, G.J. Jividen, Jr., M.G. Zwick, and V. Kumar. 2003. Chronic ulcerative stomatitis: clinical, histopathologic, and immunopathologic findings. *Oral Surg. Oral Med. Oral Pathol. Oral Radiol. Endod.* 96(6):718-726.

Souza, L.B., E.S. Andrade, M.C. Miguel, R.A. Freitas, and L.P. Pinto. 2004. Origin of stellate giant cells in oral fibrous lesions determined by immunohistochemical expression of vimentin, HHF-35, CD68 and factor XIIIa. *Pathology* 36(4):316-320.

Spiro, R.H. 1998. Verrucous carcinoma, then and now. *Am J Surg* 176(5):393-397.

Spruance, S.L., N. Bodsworth, H. Resnick, M. Conant, C. Oeuvray, J. Gao, and K. Hamed. 2006. Single-dose, patient-initiated famciclovir: a randomized, double-blind, placebo-controlled trial for episodic treatment of herpes labialis. *J. Am. Acad. Dermatol.* 55(1):47-53.

Tal, H., D. Oegiesser, and M. Tal. 2003. Gingival depigmentation by erbium:YAG laser: clinical observations and patient responses. *J. Periodontol.* 74(11):1660-1667.

Thornhill, M.H., V. Sankar, X.J. Xu, A.W. Barrett, A.S. High, E.W. Odell, P.M. Speight, and P.M. Farthing. 2006. The role of histopathological characteristics in distinguishing amalgam-associated oral lichenoid reactions and/oral lichen planus. *J Oral Pathol Med.* 35(4):233-240.

Tokgoz, B., H.I. Sari, O. Yildiz, S. Aslan, M. Sipahioglu, T. Okten, O. Oymak, and C. Utas. 2004. Effects of azithromycin on cyclosporine-induced gingival hyperplasia in renal transplant patients. *Transplant Proc.* 36(9):2699-2702.

Treister, N.S., D. Magalnick, and S.B. Woo. 2004. Oral mucosal pigmentation secondary to minocycline therapy: report of two cases and a review of the literature. *Oral Surg. Oral Med. Oral Pathol. Oral Radiol. Endod.* 97(6):718-725.

Umeda, M., and K. Shimada. 1994. Primary malignant melanoma of the oral cavity—its histological classification and treatment. *Br. J. Oral Maxillofac. Surg.* 32(1):39-47.

van der Waal, R.I., J. Buter, and I. van der Waal. 2003. Oral metastases: report of 24 cases. *Br. J. Oral Maxillofac Surg.* 41(1):3-6.

Velegraki, A., O. Nicolatou, M. Theodoridou, G. Mostrou, and N.J. Legakis. 1999. Paediatric AIDS—related linear gingival erythema: a form of erythematous candidiasis? *J. Oral Pathol. Med.* 28(4): 178-182.

Wakahara, M., T. Kiyohara, M. Kumakiri, T. Ueda, K. Ishiguro, T. Fujita, M. Amagai, and T. Hashimoto. 2005. Paraneoplastic pemphigus with widespread mucosal involvement. *Acta Derm. Venereol.* 85(6): 530-532.

Walters, J.D., J.K. Will, R.D. Hatfield, D.A. Cacchillo, and D.A. Raabe. 2001. Excision and repair of the peripheral ossifying fibroma: a report of 3 cases. *J. Periodontol.* 72(7):939-944.

Weckx, L.L., L.B. Hidal, and G. Marcucci. 1990. Oral manifestations of leukemia. *Ear Nose Throat J.* 69(5):341-342, 345-346.

Wiernik, P.H., R. De Bellis, P. Muxi, and J.P. Dutcher. 1996. Extramedullary acute promyelocytic leukemia. *Cancer* 78(12): 2510-2514.

Wine, E., A. Ballin, and I. Dalal. 2006. Infantile erythema multiforme following hepatitis B vaccine. *Acta Paediatr.* 95(7):890-891.

Wright, J.M. 1988. Intraoral melanoacanthoma: a reactive melanocytic hyperplasia. Case report. *J. Periodontol.* 59(1):53-55.

Yuan, K., L.Y. Wing, and M.T. Lin. 2002. Pathogenetic roles of angiogenic factors in pyogenic granulomas in pregnancy are modulated by female sex hormones. *J. Periodontol.* 73(7):701-708.

Zakrzewska, J.M. 1999. Fortnightly review: oral cancer. *BMJ* 318(7190): 1051-1054.

Chapter 11 Sinus Augmentation Using Tissue-Engineered Bone

Ulrike Schulze-Späte, DMD, PhD, and Luigi Montesani, MD, DDS

HISTORY

Implant placement in the edentulous maxilla often represents a clinical challenge due to insufficient bone height after crestal bone resorption and maxillary sinus pneumatization. Surgical approaches that were developed over the past years aim to restore bone height in the posterior maxilla to create a sufficient implant bed. Boyne and James (1980) were the first to describe a procedure that uses existing space in the maxillary sinus by lifting up the Schneiderian membrane from its bony surface and filling this newly created space with augmentation material. Several modifications of the originally described surgical procedure were developed; however, the basic principle of increasing maxillary bone height by placing graft material in the maxillary sinus after detaching the Schneiderian membrane remained the same (Davarpanah et al. 2001, Fugazzotto and De Paoli 2002, Summers 1994). Grafting materials used to augment bone height in the posterior maxilla can be categorized into four groups: autogenous bone, allografts (from human), xenografts (from a nonhuman species), and alloplasts (synthetic materials). Autogenous bone is the only grafting material with an osteogenic potential, and it has been shown that its use in sinus augmentation can achieve predictable results. Furthermore, autogenous bone requires shorter healing times (4 months versus 8 to 10 months) because it contains living cells and growth factors. Unfortunately, its availability is limited due to anatomical confines and donor site morbidity (Block and Kent 1997, Cammack et al. 2005, Froum et al. 1998, Garg 1999, Pikos 1996, Wheeler 1997). Several current approaches aim to overcome those boundaries; one novel approach uses concepts previously established in the field of tissue engineering. In contrast to conventional one-dimensional in vitro cell culture, tissue-engineering techniques aim to mimic an in vivo environment by using scaffolds, which arrange cells in a three-dimensional fashion (Risbud 2001). Living tissues that otherwise would be limited in their potential to grow can be contained and even expanded in vitro before being reintroduced in vivo.

Periosteum, a membrane that closely enfolds bone, consists of connective tissue and contains chondroprogenitor and osteoprogenitor cell populations (Hutmacher and Sittinger 2003). It has been shown that these progenitor cells can be isolated and stimulated in vitro to form cartilage and bone using tissue-engineering techniques (Arnold et al. 2002, Breitbart et al. 1998). In 2003, Schmelzeisen and colleagues described a clinical procedure that substitutes autogenous bone graft material with tissue-engineered bone in a sinus augmentation procedure. Periosteal tissue was harvested from the oral cavity, and its progenitor cells were isolated and expanded in a three-dimensional bioabsorbable polymer fleece matrix in vitro. The matured transplants were inserted in the maxillary sinus between the elevated Schneiderian membrane and the bony floor of the sinus. A number of follow-up publications and a prospective clinical study demonstrated successful remodeling of the graft material, thereby establishing sinus augmentation with tissue-engineered bone as a possible option for overcoming current limitations of autogenous bone grafting in the posterior maxilla (Schimming and Schmelzeisen 2004, Schmelzeisen et al. 2003).

Implant placement can occur at the same surgical appointment (immediate placement) or following a healing period (delayed placement) depending on the remaining bone height. It is generally acknowledged that for an immediate placement, at least 4 to 5 mm of remaining ridge height is necessary to achieve sufficient immobilization of implants during maturation of the sinus graft (Jensen et al. 1998).

INDICATIONS

- Insufficient bone height in the posterior maxilla for dental implant placement

- Need for a large amount of autogenous bone grafting material

- Patient's refusal to have a bone graft from a source that is not his or her own

CONTRAINDICATIONS

- Presence of uncontrolled diabetes, immune diseases, or other contraindicating systemic conditions

- Thrombocytopenia or allergically induced thrombocytopenia (type II)

- Radiation therapy to the head and neck area 12 months before proposed surgical treatment

- Chemotherapy in the 12 months before proposed surgical treatment

- Active sinus infection or a history of persistent sinus infections

- Hypersensitivity to bovine albumin, penicillin, gentamicin, amphotericin B

- Excessive smoking habit

- Alcohol and drug abuse

- Physical and psychological handicaps

- Pregnancy and lactating patients

ARMAMENTARIUM

1. For the harvesting procedure, a basic surgical kit such as the one described in *Practical Periodontal Plastic Surgery* (Dibart and Karima) and an osseous coagulum collector (Citagenix Inc., Laval, Quebec, Canada) can be used.

2. For the sinus augmentation procedure, a basic surgical kit and the following can be used:

   - Angulated elevation instruments for separation of the Schneiderian membrane from the inner bony surface of the maxillary sinus (Hu-Friedy, Chicago, IL, USA)

   - CollaTape (Zimmer Dental, Carlsbad, CA, USA)

   - Bio-Oss (Osteohealth, Shirley, NY, USA)

   - Resorbable membrane (Bio-Guide; Osteohealth; and RCM, Bicon, Boston, MA, USA)

SINUS AUGMENTATION USING TISSUE-ENGINEERED BONE DISCS

Technique

Sinus augmentation using tissue-engineered bone requires two surgical procedures: harvesting and transplant implantation surgery.

Harvesting Procedure

Periosteal tissue can be obtained from several locations in the oral cavity. However, access to the lateral cortex of the mandibular body in the apical region of the first molar area is relatively easy and not too invasive. After administering local anesthesia, an intrasulcular or intravestibular incision parallel to the mucogingival junction is made using a No. 15 blade. The incision on the buccal side of the first mandibular molar should extend at least one and one-half teeth toward the anterior and posterior in order to obtain sufficient access. A partial thickness flap is elevated to expose the underlying periosteum. After outlining the area with a No. 15 blade, the periosteal biopsy (approximately 1 cm^2) can be collected using a back action chisel or osseous coagulum collector (Fig. 11.1).

Alternatively, an alveolar bone biopsy (8 × 10 × 2 mm) can be taken from the same side or the tuberosity area after exposing the bone using a distal wedge incision. The collected tissue biopsy needs to be stored in appropriate sterile tissue containers and transferred to an in vitro cell/tissue facility for further culturing and tissue expansion. In addition, a blood sample (approximately 126 mL of blood will be sufficient for 10 tissue-engineered discs) needs to be taken from the patient. This blood sample will be used to produce serum,

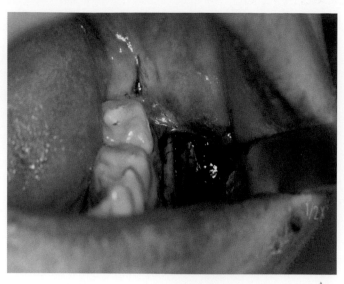

Fig. 11.1. Collection of a periosteal biopsy. Periosteal tissue was harvested from the goniac angle of the mandible.

which is essential for future culturing of the isolated periosteal cells (Schimming and Schmelzeisen 2004). The donor side can be sutured with either resorbable (5-0 chromic gut) or nonresorbable (5-0 silk) suture material.

Postoperative Management

Pain medications should be prescribed as needed. In addition, chlorhexidine rinses twice a day for 21 days starting 1 day after the surgery should be included in the postoperative regimen.

Treatment and Expansion of Periosteal Biopsies

The periosteal tissue biopsy can be cultured using a tissue engineering protocol described by Schmelzeisen and colleagues (2003). In addition, commercial companies such as Bio Tissue Technology, Freiburg, Germany, offer to overtake laborious cell culturing and provide the clinician with the finished tissue-engineered bone discs.

The periosteum needs to be enzymatically digested to isolate progenitor cells. Collagenase CLSII *(Clostridium histolyticum)* at a concentration of 333 U/mL (Biochrom, Cambridge, UK) in 1:1 DMEM/Ham's F-12 (Dulbecco's modified Eagle's medium; Invitrogen, Carlsbad, CA, USA) can be used, and the resulting cell suspension needs to be washed with phosphate-buffered saline (PBS; Invitrogen). Cells are counted using a hemocytometer and stained with Trypan blue dye to determine the overall cell viability. Afterward, they are resuspended in 1:1 DMEM/Ham's F-12 supplemented with 10% autologous serum and seeded into cell culture flasks. The

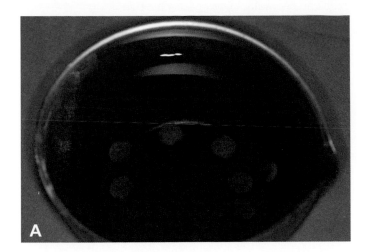
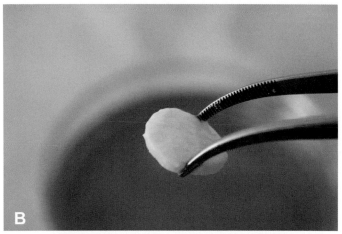

Fig. 11.2. Tissue-engineered bone discs. **A,** Discs were kept in transportation medium until implantation. **B,** Scaffolds need to be carefully handled so as to not destroy the incorporated cells.

flasks are cultured in a cell culture incubator adjusted to 37°C, 3.5% CO_2, and 95% humidity. The medium needs to be replaced every 2 days until cells reach a 70% confluency. At this point, cells are trypsinized (0.02% trypsin and 0.02% EDTA in PBS) for 5 minutes and seeded at a density of 5000/mm². This step needs to be repeated four times to increase cell number. Following trypsinization, cells are now ready to be incorporated into the transplant discs (Perka et al. 2000). Several scaffold materials such as synthetic and natural polymers, composites, and ceramics have been tested in recent years (Sittinger et al. 2004). They need to be biocompatible and resorbable to facilitate integration of the future graft into an in vivo environment. To incorporate cells into the scaffold, cells are suspended in 1:1 DMEM/Ham's and mixed with human fibrinogen (TissueColl; Baxter Immuno, Vienna, Austria) in a 3:1 ratio. The resulting cell solution is soaked into polymer fleeces (e.g., Ethicon, Cornelia, GA, USA) and subsequently polymerized by adding bovine thrombin (TissueColl) in a 1:10 PBS dilution. The transplant discs are cultured for an additional week in DMEM/Ham's supplemented with 5% autologous serum, dexamethasone 10^{-7} Mol, ß-glycerophosphate 10 mM, and ascorbic acid (50 mg/L). At this point (approximately 7 weeks after the harvesting procedure), the transplants are ready for implantation. Each final disc contains around 1.5×10^6 cells and is circa 2×10 mm in size (Fig. 11.2A, B).

TRANSPLANT IMPLANTATION SURGERY (SINUS AUGMENTATION PROCEDURE USING TISSUE-ENGINEERED BONE DISCS)

Before the sinus augmentation procedure, a computer tomography scan or panoramic radiograph should be taken from the selected area (see Fig. 11.4A later). The procedure can be performed under local anesthesia. A midcrestal incision is made with mesial and distal releasing incisions extending well into the buccal fold. The mucoperiosteal flap is reflected in a full-thickness manner, and care needs to be taken to completely release the tissue for a tension-free access to the lateral wall of the maxillary sinus.

There are three classic approaches to enter the maxillary sinus. In the Caldwell-Luc approach, the window is anterior to the zygomatic buttress; in a low position, the window is situated next to the alveolar crest; and in a mid maxillary position, the lateral window is situated between alveolar crest and zygomatic buttress (Lazzara 1996, Summers 1994, Zitzmann and Scharer 1998). In the above-introduced application, a lateral window approach is recommended. However, in any case, the osteotomy window should be placed according to the anatomical structure of the maxillary sinus and its inferior horizontal border should be 3 to 4 mm above the sinus floor. The oval window is outlined under continuous sterile saline irrigation with a high-speed handpiece and either a carbide or a diamond bur (Fig. 11.3A). As an alternative, piezoelectric surgery could be used, reducing the risks of underlying membrane perforation (Vercellotti et al. 2001). The bone covering the window can either be thinned uniformly all around or in a trap door manner, which uses the superior border as a hinge (Fig. 11.3B).

In both techniques, the bony window is carefully pushed inward and at the same time the Schneiderian membrane is detached from its underlying bony surface using angulated elevation instruments. Attention should be paid to preserving the integrity of the sinus membrane by keeping elevation instruments in constant contact with the internal bony sinus wall during the membrane elevation process. After elevation, membrane integrity can be checked with the Valsalva maneuver (El Charkawi et al. 2005). Occurring tears can be repaired. For small tears (less than 5 mm), a fast resorbing collagen membrane such as Collatape (Zimmer Dental, Carlsbad, CA, USA) can be used to cover the tear. Repair of larger perforations requires a more rigid and longer-lasting membrane (Biomend; Zimmer Dental) (Zimbler et al. 1998). In

cases of major membrane destruction, it is recommended to abort the grafting procedure and wait 6 to 9 months for membrane regeneration (Berengo et al. 2004). It is important to detach the membrane sufficiently from its walls because it has been shown that in an adequately elevated membrane, tears can heal without complications.

In contrast, lacerations could remain open in membranes that are stretched too much (Jensen et al. 1998). In addition, insufficient membrane elevation might subsequently result in a graft that is not adequate in its dimensions to support future implants. In particular, the medial and anterior walls are common regions to display insufficient grafting. Therefore, grafting the anterior wall first is a habit many surgeons developed to prevent this problem. Furthermore, it is advised that the clinician holds up the membrane with a periosteal elevator while packing the bone graft against the medial wall to prevent packing against a Schneiderian membrane that has "come down" as a result of patient's breathing. It also should be kept in mind that the ostium that represents the connection between the middle meatus of the nose and the maxillary sinus

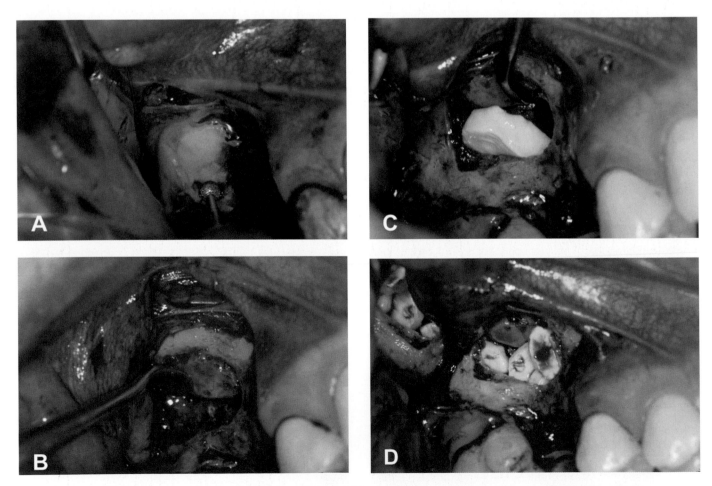

Fig. 11.3. Sinus augmentation using tissue-engineered bone discs. **A,** A lateral window was outlined to access the maxillary sinus. **B,** The Schneiderian membrane was elevated from its bony surface to create space for the augmentation material. **C, D,** Tissue-engineered bone discs were implanted into the maxillary sinus.

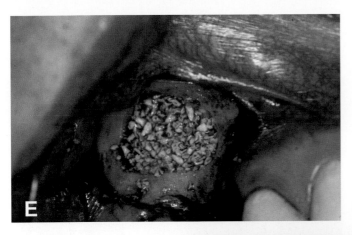

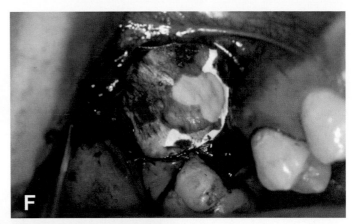

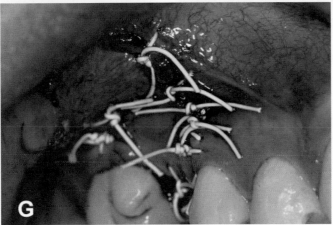

Fig. 11.3. (*continued*) **E,** The discs were covered with BioOss (Osteohealth) augmentation material (optional). **F,** The grafted area was covered with a resorbable membrane (Bioguide; Osteohealth). **G,** The flap was sutured in its original position with single interrupted sutures (Gore-Tex; Gore Medical).

is approximately 25 mm above the floor of the sinus. Blockade due to extensive sinus grafting can result in a chronic infection of the maxillary sinus (Doud Galli et al. 2001).

Assuming that the membrane is elevated sufficiently, the tissue-engineered discs, which can be kept in the transportation medium during the procedure, are then inserted into the sinus and gently packed until the space between the sinus membrane and bony walls of the sinus is filled (Fig. 11.3C, D). In addition, bone augmentation material such as BioOss (Osteohealth, Shirley, NY, USA) can be used as a protective layer on the outside of the graft (Fig. 11.3E). The window should be covered with a membrane that overlaps its outlines and thereby protects the grafted side. Either a nonresorbable membrane with securing tacks or a resorbable one can be used for this purpose (Fig. 11.3F).

Afterward, the mucoperiosteal flap is positioned back to cover the surgical site. It might be necessary to release the periosteum of the flap with a No. 15 blade in order to facili-

tate a tension-free closure. The flap can now be sutured with either resorbable (such as Vicryl; Ethicon, Carnelia, GA, USA) or nonresorbable (such as Gore-Tex suture; Gore Medical, Flagstaff, AZ, USA) suture material in single interrupted sutures (Fig. 11.3G). Whenever necessary, these sutures can be replaced by a continuous suture and further secured with horizontal mattress sutures.

Postoperative Management

- Antibiotic therapy should be started the day before the procedure: 500 mg amoxicillin 3 times daily for 7 days (300 mg clindamycin 4 times daily should be prescribed for penicillin-sensitive patients).

- *Analgesics:* Acetaminophen plus codeine (Tylenol #3) or ibuprofen (Motrin 600 mg) 3 times a day or as necessary is recommended.

- *Anti-inflammatory drugs:* Dexamethasone can be prescribed for 5 days in the following manner (day of surgery:

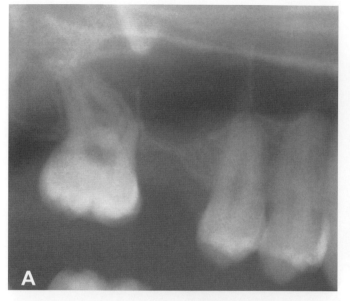

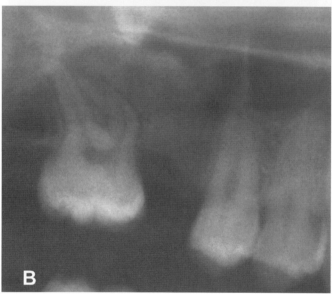

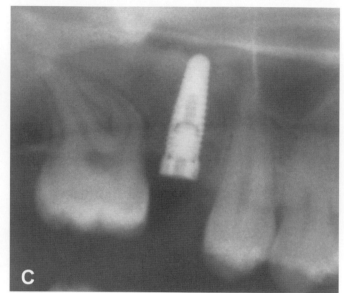

Fig. 11.4 Radiographic evaluation of the grafted site. **A,** A periapical radiograph was taken and revealed inadequate bone height before implant placement. **B,** Radiograph depicting the augmented site before implant placement. **C,** Implant was placed successfully in the grafted site achieving primary stability.

3.75 mg; day 2: 3 mg; day 3: 2.25 mg: day 4: 1.5 mg; day 5: 0.75 mg). This will control the swelling and alleviate the discomfort.

- *Afrin spray:* Patients should be given this spray to use so they will not blow their nose for 2 weeks, as that will impair proper healing of the graft.

- *Antiseptic rinses:* Chlorhexidine digluconate rinses twice a day for 21 days starting 1 day after the surgery are recommended.

- Patients can wear their complete dentures after the procedure; however, the buccal flange needs to be reduced and later on relined with a soft reliner. Partial dentures should be worn only if they have an acrylic base, which allows ap-

propriate relief and facilitates soft relining. However, it is recommended to advise the patient that the denture is worn for aesthetic reasons and not for function until the day of suture removal.

Healing

Studies revealed sufficient new bone formation 4 months after implantation of the tissue-engineered bone discs (Schmelzeisen et al. 2003). Therefore, dental implants can be placed 4 months after the grafting procedure (Fig. 11.4B, C). A core biopsy can be taken during the surgery and subjected to histologic staining to determine current mineralization status of the augmented bone (Fig. 11.5). Afterward, implants can be restored according to standard protocols (Fig. 11.6).

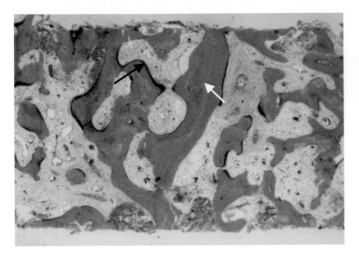

Fig. 11.5 Histologic staining of core biopsy taken from the future implant side. Goldner's staining shows mineralized bone (green; see *white arrow*) and newly formed osteoid (red; see *black arrow*).

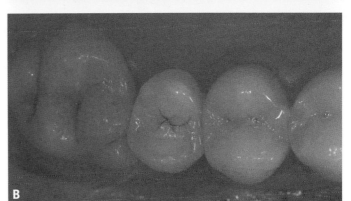

Fig. 11.6 Clinical view of the restored implant. **A, B.** Implant was restored with a single porcelain-fused metal (PFM) crown.

Possible Complications

Complications occurring after sinus augmentation with tissue-engineered bone should not be different from complications associated with other grafting materials, assuming that the discs were prepared and transported under sterile conditions.

Swelling, Bruising, and Bleeding

Patients might experience swelling and bruising in the surgical areas after the procedures. It is recommended that cold pads be used for the initial 24 hours. Afterward, the application of warm pads in combination with anti-inflammatory medications will help to reduce swelling and discomfort. It is not unusual for patients to report an exacerbated feeling of pain 5 days after the procedure because at this time point the corticosteroid regimen has ended. Therefore, patients should be informed beforehand and advised to continue taking the nonsteroidal anti-inflammatory drugs for 1 week.

In the case of nasal bleeding due to laceration of the Schneiderian membrane, patients should be reassured (as this will happen after they have left your office) and pressure with a cotton ball should be applied to stop the nasal bleeding.

Infraorbital Nerve Paresthesia

Paresthesia of the area innervated by the infraorbital nerve can be caused by blunt retraction over the neurovascular bundle. It usually is transient and disappears within a few weeks. However, in some cases, long-lasting paresthesia, up to several months, is possible.

Infection of the Grafted Site and Membrane Exposure

Infection spreading from an infected graft can lead to pansinusitis, can spread to the orbit, dura, and brain, and requires intervention. An early sign is the occurrence of an intraoral swelling 1 week postsurgery; however, signs of infections can be detected as early as 3 days. In the case of an infection, prescription of antibiotics such as clindamycin with a loading dose of 600 mg followed by a dosage of 300 mg 4 times is recommended. Metronidazole can be added for anaerobic coverage at 500 mg 3 times daily. Usually, localized infections will respond to the treatment. However, in case of persistent symptomatology, it is imperative to pursue aggressive treatment, which includes incision and drainage over the original incision line. In addition, aerobic and anaerobic culture results could be used as a supportive adjunct to determine future treatment.

Sometimes local debridement is appropriate and sufficient. If the graft needs to be completely removed, a long-lasting collagen membrane should be used to cover the window. After a healing period of 3 to 4 months, the site can be reentered for an additional grafting procedure. In response to an infection, oroantral fistulas can form that are treatable with antibiotics and oral chlorhexidine rinses. Nevertheless, large and persistent fistulas require surgical intervention. In case of a premature exposure of the membrane, it has been shown that oral bacteria can penetrate the membrane surface within 4 weeks (Simion et al. 1994). Thus, it is advised to continue the use of chlorhexidine mouth rinses until the final implant surgery. In any case, the patient should be closely followed in order to intervene if an infection develops and the membrane needs to be removed.

Taken together, infection should be treated in a comprehensive way to minimize the risk of spreading and maximize the success of the grafting procedure.

REFERENCES

Arnold, U., K. Lindenhayn, and C. Perka. 2002. In vitro-cultivation of human periosteum derived cells in bioresorbable polymer-TCP-composites. *Biomaterials* 23:2303–2310.

Berengo, M., S. Sivolella, Z. Majzoub, and G. Cordioli. 2004. Endoscopic evaluation of the bone-added osteotome sinus floor elevation procedure. *Int. J. Oral Maxillofac. Surg.* 33(2):189–194.

Block, M.S., and Kent J.N. 1997. Sinus augmentation for dental implants: the use of autogenous bone. *J. Oral Maxillofac. Surg.* 55(11):1281–1286.

Boyne, P.J., and R.A. James. 1980. Grafting of the maxillary sinus floor with autogenous marrow and bone. *J. Oral Surg.* 38(8):613–616.

Breitbach, A.S., D.A. Grande, R. Kessler, J.T. Ryabi, R.J. Fitzsimmons, and R.T. Grant. 1998. Tissue engineered bone repair of calvarial defects using culture periosteal cells. *Plast. Reconstr. Surg.* 101:567–574.

Cammack, G.V. 2nd., M. Nevins, D.S. Clem 3rd., J.P. Hatch, and J.T. Mellonig. 2005. Histologic evaluation of mineralized and demineralized freeze-dried bone allograft for ridge and sinus augmentations. *Int. J. Periodont. Restor. Dent.* 25(3):231–237.

Davarpanah, M., H. Martinez, J.F. Tecucianu, G. Hage, and R. Lazzara. 2001. The modified osteotome technique. *Int. J. Periodont. Restor. Dent.* 21(6):599–607.

Dibart, S., and M. Karima. 2006. *Practical Periodontal Plastic Surgery.* Blackwell Publishing, Ames, IA.

Doud Galli, S.K., R.A. Lebowitz, R.J. Giacchi, R. Glickman, and J.B. Jacobs. 2001. Chronic sinusitis complicating sinus lift surgery. *Am. J. Rhinol.* 15(3):181–186.

El Charkawi, H.G., A.S. El Askary, and A. Ragab. 2005. Endoscopic removal of an implant from the maxillary sinus: a case report. *Implant Dent.* 14(1):30–35.

Froum, S.J., D.P. Tarnow, S.S. Wallace, M.D. Rohrer, and S.C. Cho. 1998. Sinus floor elevation using an organic bovine bone matrix (OsteoGraf/N) with and without autogenous bone: a clinical, histologic, radiographic, and histomorphometric analysis—part 2 of an ongoing prospective study. *Int. J. Periodont. Restor. Dent.* 18(6):528-543.

Fugazzotto, P.A., and S. De Paoli. 2002. Sinus floor augmentation at the time of maxillary molar extraction: success and failure rates of 137 implants in function for up to 3 years. *J. Periodontol.* 73(1):39-44.

Garg, A.K. 1999. Augmentation grafting of the maxillary sinus for placement of dental implants: anatomy, physiology, and procedures. *Implant Dent.* 8(1):36-46.

Hutmacher, D.W., and M. Sittinger. 2003. Periosteal cells in bone tissue engineering. *Tiss. Eng.* 9(Suppl 1):S45-S64.

Jensen, O.T., L.B. Shulman, M.S. Block, and V.J. Iacono. 1998. Report of the Sinus Consensus Conference of 1996. *Int. J. Oral Maxillofac. Implants* 13(Suppl):11-45.

Lazzara, R.J. 1996. The sinus elevation procedure in endosseous implant therapy. *Curr. Opin. Periodontol.* 3:178-183.

Perka, C., O. Schultz, R.S. Spitzer, K. Lindenhayn, G.R. Burmester, and M. Sittinger. 2000. Segmental bone repair by tissue-engineered periosteal cell transplants with bioresorbable fleece and fibrin scaffolds in rabbits. *Biomaterials* 21(11):1145-1153.

Pikos, M.A. 1996. Chin grafts as donor sites for maxillary bone augmentation—part II. *Dental Implantol. Update* 7(1):1-4.

Risbud, M. 2001. Tissue engineering: implications in the treatment of organ and tissue defects. *Biogerontology* 2:117-125.

Schmelzeisen, R., R. Schimming, and M. Sittinger. 2003. Making bone: implant insertion into tissue-engineered bone for maxillary sinus floor augmentation—a preliminary report. *J. Craniomaxillofac. Surg.* 31:34-39.

Schimming, R., and R. Schmelzeisen. 2004. Tissue-engineered bone for maxillary sinus augmentation. *J. Oral Maxillofac. Surg.* 62(6):724-729.

Sittinger, M., D.W. Hutmacher, and M.V. Risbud. 2004. Current strategies for cell delivery in cartilage and bone regeneration. *Curr. Opin. Biotechnol.* 15(5):411-418.

Simion, M., P. Trisi, M. Maglione, and A. Piattelli. 1994. A preliminary report on a method for studying the permeability of expanded polytetrafluoroethylene membrane to bacteria in vitro: a scanning electron microscopic and histological study. *J. Periodontol.* 65(8):755-761.

Summers, R.B. 1994. A new concept in maxillary implant surgery: the osteotome technique. *Compend. Cont.g Educ. Dent.* 15(2):152, 154-156.

Vercellotti, T., S. De Paoli, and M. Nevins. 2001. The piezoelectric bony window osteotomy and sinus membrane elevation: introduction of a new technique for simplification of the sinus augmentation procedure. *Int. J. Periodont. Restor. Dent.* 21(6):561-567.

Wheeler, S.L. 1997. Sinus augmentation for dental implants: the use of alloplastic materials. *J. Oral Maxillofac. Surg.* 55(11):1287-1293.

Zimbler, M.S., R.A. Lebowitz, R. Glickman, L.E. Brecht,and J.B. Jacobs. 1998. Antral augmentation, osseointegration, and sinusitis: the otolaryngologist's perspective. *Am. J. Rhinol.* 12(5):311-316.

Zitzmann, N.U., and P. Scharer. 1998. Sinus elevation procedures in the resorbed posterior maxilla. Comparison of the crestal and lateral approaches. *Oral Surg. Oral Med. Oral Pathol. Oral Radiol. Endod.* 85(1):8-17.

Index